Salt

Dr. Matt Klingler PT, DPT, OCS

&

Dr. Erik Gullen PT, DPT

CONTENTS

ACKNOWLEDGMENTS

We would like to thank our amazing staff here at Village for their desire to learn and grow, our clients for giving us inspiration every day, Carmen Singleton for taking stellar photos, Mark Miller for his editing prowess, Ethan Bailey for designing the slick cover, and our wives, Nicole and Krissy, for being the amazing women they are.

Dr. Matt Klingler | Dr. Erik Gullen

INTRODUCTION

Salubrious

adjective
health-giving; healthy.

That's it. You can now define *salubrious*.

My grandfather used to say, "If everyday you learn just one new word, eventually you will be the smartest person in the world." By trade he was a journalist, so words were his business. He knew that the right word at the right time could make all the difference. So right now, if you only read the first page of this book, you can at least say you are on your way to becoming the smartest person in the world.

But I hope that you continue reading. I believe that if you do, you will not only be able to define *salubrious*, but it may come to define *you*.

So where did this strange word come from? Its origin is the Latin *salus*, meaning "health." Also sharing this Latin origin is the Spanish word *salud*, which you may have heard shouted cheerfully before toasting cervezas or tequila! In English *salubrious* was most often used to describe an environment. However, over the course of the 19th century, its mention faded. Coincidence or not, it shares an uncanny, inverse relationship with the Industrial Revolution.

While a full discussion on the Industrial Revolution is beyond the scope of this book, most folks are familiar with it as a time when the human environment changed rapidly and dramatically. Think assembly lines, slaughterhouses, and factories. Think Oliver Twist. Think smokestacks, chemical wastes, and machines that build machines that build machines. Think mass production, mass marketing, and mass transit.

Our environment changed, and so did our health. To be fair, many technological developments were helpful, such as the mass production and distribution of vaccines for pathogenic diseases like polio and tuberculosis. Once great epidemics, they are now all but eliminated from modern populations. Unfortunately, we have also developed a whole new category of epidemic: metabolic disease. Metabolic diseases are things like obesity, type II diabetes, and hypertension — you know, the stuff that happens when you sit around and eat too much junk food!

But it's bigger than that. The technological advancements of the Industrial Revolution gave way to a snowball of trade-offs.

We gained the ability to produce great quantities of food, but lost the quality of those foods by exhausting the soil of its nutrients and modifying them to increase shelf life.

We gained the ability to eat anytime we wanted, as much as we wanted, but lost the simple appreciation and knowledge to tend a garden and prepare a home-cooked meal for our family.

We gained the ability to travel great distances of land, air, and sea, but lost the practice of walking through a forest or riding on horseback.

We gained great knowledge and appreciation of the natural environment in sciences such as geology, biology, etc., but have left it polluted and often uninhabitable.

Humans have always faced the same fundamental temptations and pitfalls: greed, laziness, impatience, arrogance, and so on. We have also had the same desires: to be healthy, good stewards, responsible, happy, connected. In the old environment, there was space for these merits. In the modern environment, we are boxed in, cut off, unable to find room to shape the environment around us for good. It often seems we are too far gone. And so many of us give up and give in.

Macro-control: There are some things about our environment we cannot change. We cannot individually change the air quality in LA, the relative price and availability of nourishing food to junk food, nor the demands of LA's never-sleeping economy on our jobs and careers.

Micro-Control: There are some things in our environments over which we have total control. We have control over the direction we are headed. We have control over how we respond to circumstances.

For everything we cannot control in the environment around us, there are a few key things we can — and must!

We do not exist in isolation, but in context and community — in an environment. That environment can be a wasteland or a vibrant garden, and we are smart enough to shape it either way.

Like needles in haystacks, there are still salubrious microenvironments. To find them you need to know what you are looking for. You need knowledge — a solid primer for the *whats* and *hows* of human movement and nourishment. You also need to know who you are looking for — small, well-educated, and highly-motivated groups of healthy rebels who still believe that living fully is possible — peers, mentors, coaches, and experts that can keep each other encouraged, accountable, and connected. The *who* is just as important as the *what*.

Salubrious is your guide to reshaping your environment to promote the three key elements of wellness: moving often, moving well, and eating well.

In this book, we propose a call back to eating the way our ancestors ate, to moving often and in the ways we were created to move.

This book is a starting point. We hope that you will read it and take to heart the core principles of moving well, moving often, and eating well. But more importantly, we hope that it will open your eyes to recognize all types of environments: both those that give health and those that steal it. If you can develop the skill of placing yourself in salubrious environments, many difficult-to-control facets of your health and wellness will take care of themselves. Ultimately, if you are reading this and find yourself near us, we hope that you will stop by our little environment. We hope that you will be a part of the story that is unfolding.

Life is meant to be lived to the fullest. Life is meant to be salubrious.

Dr. Matt Klingler | Dr. Erik Gullen

PART 1: COMMUNICATE WELL THROUGH FOOD

Dr. Matt Klingler | Dr. Erik Gullen

We humans were designed with everything we need already built into our genetic code to be healthy.

Our genes need the right environment and good nutritional and movement communication so they can do what they were designed to do.

Sunflowers thrive in warm weather. With nutrient-rich soil and appropriate watering, they will grow big, a vibrant yellow, and beautiful. But even in suboptimal conditions, they will survive and bloom. However, they will never reach their full potential. Over time, if left in a poor environment, the sunflower will wither and die.

We humans are the same as the sunflower. We can survive for 60-plus years in a poor nutritional environment, but we certainly won't thrive.

When we consider food as simply a mathematical formula of calories in vs. calories out, it degrades our understanding of the effect of food on our body.

Although calories are important, food is more like a language that communicates with the cells and DNA of our body to produce health or disease.

With movements like Low-fat, Atkins, "If It Fits Your Macros", and Weight Watchers, our culture has become obsessed with calories, points, and macronutrients. Weight loss and health are seen as simply eating less and moving more.

A recent study in the Journal of the American Medical Association found that people who eat a diet low in processed carbohydrates, vegetable oils, and sugar lost weight even without focusing on caloric intake.[1] The participants in the study focused on eating a diet rich in whole foods and vegetables. In other words, they created a good environment for nutritional communication for their bodies.

When we eat inflammatory foods, like sugar and vegetable oil, they cause increased levels of systemic inflammation in our body.

Diseases like heart disease stem from long-term inflammatory changes inside the vessels of our heart.

Therefore, it's imperative we eat a diet rich in anti-inflammatory foods like leafy green vegetables (or, heck, any vegetable for that matter), healthy fats like grass-fed butter, free-range meats, and avocados.

We also need to eat food from good sources. We need to become educated consumers who understand where our food comes from and how it was produced.

A comprehensive dietary education is one of the most powerful forms of preventative medicine.

With *Salubrious*, it's our mission to educate and equip you with the tools to create understanding of how to communicate well with your body through the food you eat.

At Village Fitness, we teach our clients how to communicate well with their bodies through food. We break up nutritional communication into digestible habits. Generally, we will work on each habit for a month before moving on to another habit.

In Part 1, we will explore each habit in depth.

Here's to you living salubriously and creating an environment of health through the food you eat.

---

[1] "Effect of Low-Fat vs Low-Carbohydrate Diet on ... - The JAMA Network." 20 Feb. 2018, https://jamanetwork.com/journals/jama/fullarticle/2673150. Accessed 25 Sep. 2018.

CHAPTER 1: INFLAMMATION

"I've been trying to lose weight for the last year. At first, I was successful. I lost 30 pounds in the first 6 months. But now, I still have a lot more weight to lose and the scale won't budge. What gives?"

If you're seemingly doing all the right things with your diet and exercise while trying to lose weight and the scale isn't moving, it can be very frustrating. The answer may be inflammation.

I've consulted with many folks who have started exercising and lowering their calories only to wind up far from their weight-loss goals and frustrated with their progress. I'll hear things like "I need to get my thyroid checked," or "It's impossible for women to lose weight during menopause."

While thyroid levels and menopausal hormone changes can certainly impact weight loss, inflammation usually plays a bigger role.

In fact, many of the chronic health, pain, and weight problems plaguing our society are the result of inflammatory changes from a poor diet.

Not all inflammation is bad. In fact, if we get injured with a paper cut, we want the inflammatory process to occur in order to bring healing and antibacterial agents to the surface of our skin. Once the cut is healed, inflammation subsides because its job is done.

If I see a patient in my clinical practice with new swelling in their knee, I'll congratulate them that their healing response is functioning well. Inflammation protects, heals, and fights infections. Without inflammation we would have a tough time surviving.

In a normal and healthy body, inflammation is important and

useful. With dietary imbalance, however, inflammation is not a temporary problem solver but rather a permanent burden. This creates issues like disturbed cellular growth and makes us more likely to become the victim of diseases such as cancer, heart disease, and diabetes.

Inflammation has also been linked to diseases like chronic pain, fibromyalgia, and arthritis.[2]

When the body is in a state of inflammation, it is quite difficult to burn fat as fuel and build lean tissue such as muscle, nerves, and bones.

Inflammation may be the biggest hindrance standing between you and a lean, healthy, pain-free body.

In Latin the word inflammation means "to set on fire." You can imagine chronic, systemic inflammation in the body like a slow-burning fire smoldering inside your body. It's often subtle enough that we don't feel the effects, but the long-term consequences of unchecked inflammation are catastrophic.

Yes, this is something to be feared.

If you have inflammation in your joints, it can cause joint pain. In the stomach, inflammation can cause nausea and cramping. Inflammation causes irritability, hormonal issues, weight gain, and chronic fatigue. It prevents our body from building muscle and makes it more challenging to burn fat as fuel.

In the medical world, these problems often get pegged as a normal part of old age, a result of bad genetics, stress, or being overweight. People are given pills to pacify the symptoms, but the root cause is not addressed and the fire continues to burn.

Rarely does the medical community talk about dietary inflammation. Just look at the meals we feed patients in the hospital who are fighting off infections or recovering from surgery. They are mainly processed carbs, vegetable oil, and sugar-laden juices.

At Village, we believe these problems are NOT a normal part of the aging process but rather a manifestation of poor communication between your food and your body.

Inflammation is truculent. It obstructs the natural communication between our cells and makes us store fat more

---

[2] "Effect and Treatment of Chronic Pain in Inflammatory Arthritis." https://www.ncbi.nlm.nih.gov/pmc/articles/PMC3552517/. Accessed 25 Sep. 2018.

readily. As we will talk about in the next chapter, instead of looking at calories, we need to think of the words our food is communicating.

How Most People Try To Lose Weight

When most folks set out to lose weight, they try to do so by eating a little less of the same pro-inflammatory foods that got them into the dire situation they are in to begin with.

This may temporarily cause weight loss (like dropping calories low), but it does not solve the long-term issues wreaking havoc inside your body.

With clients, I used to address problems like systemic inflammation long after we'd gotten a client eating a low-calorie diet. Now, however, an anti-inflammatory diet is one of the first things we tackle.

Diets high in vegetable oil and sugar are so damaging to things like artery walls, brain cells, and our skin that the body has to initiate the inflammatory response to heal when we ingest foods like these. In the short term, this is fine. But chronically it leads to many of the life-altering diseases we seek to avoid.

Inflammation even has an impact on our ability to build muscle. When we can't build muscle, it slows the metabolism and makes weight loss difficult.

So, How Do You Quell Inflammation In The Body?

1. Stop eating inflammatory vegetable oils like canola.

2. Keep your sugar intake low. This means eating more vegetables instead of fruits and even keeping your carbs a bit lower. Eating fewer carbs helps make more room for leafy greens and healthy fats.

3. Eat plenty of healthy fats. These include animal fats like those found in egg yolks and meat.

4. Eat a plethora of vegetables in a wide bandwidth (lots of variety).

We will go over all of these in depth in later chapters.

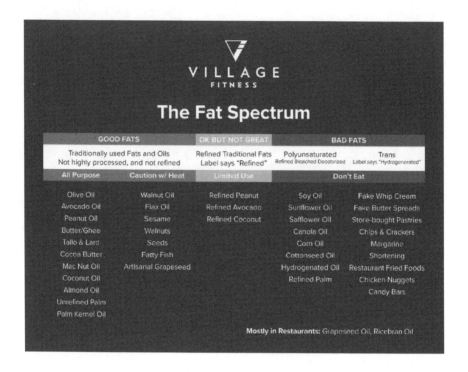

The Twinkie Diet

Processed food is ubiquitous and difficult to avoid in our culture.

In undergrad we learned about something called the Twinkie Diet.

A professor at Kansas State University set out to lose weight by eating a low-calorie diet comprised of nothing but Twinkies and processed foods. Over the course of 2 months, he lost 27 pounds and saw a decrease in his LDL (bad cholesterol) and an increase in his HDL (good cholesterol).[3]

I share this story not to encourage you to eat whatever you want or to show that it's all about calories in vs. calories out. Rather, I share this to illustrate that **any** diet can lead to weight loss.

BUT many diets don't address the root cause of the problem, which is poor nutritional communication. Yes, you may lose weight

---

[3] "Twinkie diet helps nutrition professor lose 27 pounds - CNN.com."
http://www.cnn.com/2010/HEALTH/11/08/twinkie.diet.professor/index.html.
Accessed 25 Sep. 2018.

in the short term, like our Kansas State University professor, but will you stay lean and healthy long-term? Not a chance.

Trying to reverse the inflammation by simply eating fewer of the pro-inflammatory foods will yield weight loss. But, as you may have found out, it's temporary and difficult to sustain.

Worse yet, the systemic inflammation is still there. And the systemic inflammation is the real culprit for many of the chronic diseases our society suffers from today.

A Diet, You Say?

Once upon a time, our great-great-great-grandparents ate a diet rich with good nutritional communication. Every day, they moved often, grew their own vegetables, made their own grain, and killed their own meat. The lived off the land and were healthy because of it.

Then along came the Industrial Revolution, the rise of processed food, and technology.

Now Americans are more sedentary and unhealthy than ever before. Even with medicine advancing constantly, we are still suffering from chronic diseases like diabetes and heart disease. People are living longer but not living well.

At Village, we believe we need to return to eating the way our ancestors ate. We need to eat a diet rich in anti-inflammatory vegetables, healthy fats, and protein. We need to get away from the relatively newly-introduced foods containing processed carbs, sugar, and vegetable oil.

Is This Diet Low-Carb?

In short, yes.

Carbs raise our blood sugar, promote inflammation when we eat too many, and make weight loss challenging. If we eat carbs in abundance, it can actually damage our metabolism and make it more challenging for us to burn fat as fuel. More than 100 to 150 grams of carbs per day can wreak havoc on our metabolism. We will cover this in depth in Chapter 3.

Fat Makes You Fat, Right?

Natural fats are rarely the culprit of weight gain. It's actually difficult to gain weight when eating a diet higher in natural fats. In fact, a diet low in fat makes it difficult to burn fat as fuel and makes weight loss more challenging.

Can I Never Eat Sugar Or Eat Out Again?

After reading about inflammation, it can make you feel like you should never eat a meal out, eat ice cream, or have a glass of Prosecco.

What I am proposing is not a life of neurotic food perfectionism. I would hate to see people become consumed by never putting anything toxic inside their bodies. I want you to have balance.

You don't want to be the person who brings their own food in Tupperware to a dinner party. Trust me, those people aren't cool.

I do firmly believe we need to be eating an anti-inflammatory diet most (nearly all) of the time. Then, when you want to have ice cream, enjoy a meal at your favorite barbeque place, or eat with friends, just do it. Enjoy it slowly and then get back to the patterns of eating in a way that communicates well with your body.

The important piece to the equation is intentionality. Know which foods communicate poorly with your body.

The food you eat should communicate well with your body most of the time. If you want a number, I would say 90% of your meals should be "healthy." This means eating meals rich in anti-inflammatory vegetables and healthy fats and absent of sugar and vegetable oil. This means paying attention to where your foods came from, what your food ate, and how it is prepared.

This means living life intentionally and creating an environment where you and your body can thrive.

Rachel

When Rachel and I met, she told me she had been on every diet known to man (and a few not known). They all worked temporarily but were unsustainable. She was frustrated and understandably skeptical that our program could ever work for someone like her.

We started talking about inflammation and its role in the body. She committed to give the anti-inflammatory diet a try. She eliminated vegetable oils and replaced her low-fat yogurt with an organic, grass-fed, full-fat variety. She loaded up on vegetables and meat from good sources. She kept her carbohydrate intake low.

Then she saw results.

To date, she has lost over 25 pounds. She doesn't feel hungry or like she's on a diet. She feels energetic and 10 years younger. She feels salubrious.

Rachel has learned to communicate well with her body through the food she eats.

CHAPTER 2: STOP COUNTING CALORIES

Ganesh

I sat across the table from Ganesh, one of my first personal training clients.

"I don't get it, Matt. I'm still eating just like I was before and I've started to gain weight," he said.

All I knew at the time to help people lose weight was calories in vs. calories out. So we cut calories and kept a food journal.

And by golly, it worked!

Ganesh lost a few pounds each week, losing over 70 pounds in our first year together.

Then, just after getting under 200 pounds, his weight loss stopped. Within a few months, he had gained a few of the pounds back. After a few years, all the weight came back and then some.

I was really frustrated. He was the first major weight-loss success of any of my clients, and he gained the weight back.

Looking back, I can see the problem was in the foundation we set. I didn't set him up for success long-term by equipping him with the tools needed to see long-term progress.

I, like most of modern medicine, gave him only what he needed to fix the symptoms of being overweight, not the cause.

So, armed with his food journal and reduced-calorie diet, he dutifully ate less and lost weight. He lost weight simply by eating a little less of the inflammatory and toxic foods he was already eating. And like I mentioned earlier, it works temporarily.

But we never fixed the root cause. I never taught him how to communicate with his body through the food he was eating.

Why We Can't Start With Calories

Whether or not we gain or lose weight is less about calories in and out and more about how our food and movement communicate with our bodies. Food is a language that guides the cells of our body.

One of the major reasons diets fail is that people cut calories but don't give a thought to the communication of inflammatory sugar, processed food, and toxic fats they are still pumping into their body.

Your body will go into panic mode as it realizes you are depriving it of the nutrients it needs to survive. When given a slight chance to store energy as fat, it will do its absolute best. Stem cells will be ready and willing to convert into fat cells in an environment like this.

When we instead get folks eating a salubrious diet and moving often and well, their stem cells are in an environment where they can turn into more useful tissue like blood vessel, bone, muscle, or nerve.

There is much more to weight loss and health than calories in vs. calories out. We have to see our foods as more than simple fuel, nutrients, carbs, protein, fat, and vitamins.

Calories are important. There is merit and value to tracking the food you eat, as we will see in the Food Journaling chapter. But until you understand and implement good nutritional communication, all the food journaling and calorie counting in the world will be a waste.

Food is a language of communication between the environment where it came from (the ground, ocean, forest) and the environment of our cells.

You can think of it as "eating nature," if that's not too far out in left field.

I remember the first time I had truly fresh seafood. I was in Haiti on a beach, and a man pulled up in his rowboat, having just caught fresh oysters. They were AMAZING! I could taste the salt of the seawater and the freshness of the oyster. Similarly, the deep yellowy-orange color of an egg yolk from a free-range chicken tells us a story about the life the chicken lived. You can taste the difference, too.

In my undergraduate exercise science degree and even in my doctoral program, we were taught a simple formula for weight loss.

Calories eaten — calories burned = weight loss or gain.

When I started as a personal trainer, I would sit down and lay out the above formula.

Some people lost weight.

Yet I couldn't shake the fact that many of the clients I worked with still struggled to lose weight even though they were sticking under their calorie goals.

"Matt, I work out, I eat 1600 calories a day like you told me to, and I've hit a plateau. What's going on?"

I chalked it up to thyroid levels, wrecked metabolisms, and clients not being altogether truthful about what they were eating.

But I was missing something.

You see, food is far more than simple fuel. It's a language communicating with every single cell in our body.

If you've been gaining weight or struggling to lose, it's because you've been eating foods that communicate in a way that tells your body to gain or maintain weight.

The output of a lean, healthy physique — or an unhealthy and overweight one — depends largely on how we communicate with our body.

To see this difference played out, let's take a look at two essential fatty acids: omega 6 fatty acids and omega 3 fatty acids. These are nearly identical. However, to our cells they are antithetical.

In the 90s a journalist named Joe Robinson interviewed a PhD candidate who was studying the astounding cellular process of apoptosis (cell suicide). He discovered that when he injected omega 3 into rats with tumors, it slowed and even reversed the rats' cancer cell growth. However, when he injected omega 6, it accelerated the cancer cell growth fourfold.[4]

These two types of fats contain nearly identical chemical energy. So why would one tell cells to multiply and the other to divide and delete?

Sources of omega 3 fats include eggs, cold water fatty fish, and plants like flax.

---

[4] "Effect of omega-3 fatty acids on the progression of metastases after the ...." https://www.ncbi.nlm.nih.gov/pubmed/9816126. Accessed 25 Sep. 2018.

Sources of omega 6 are tough to avoid and include vegetable oils like canola and sunflower oil, corn, soy, and animals that are fed these things.

Don't miss the main point: We don't simply need less omega 6 and more omega 3.

"Our cells are attuned to the nature of the chemical messages we send them every time we eat."[5] - Catherine Shanahan, *Deep Nutrition*

We can create an environment where cells are more likely to mutate and turn cancerous or one where they are more likely to thrive.

What's key to being healthy is eating foods that send the right messages.

The formula for weight loss and health, then, is simple:

Eliminate foods that promote inflammation and block cellular communication like sugar and vegetable oils. Eat foods that create an environment in your body to build healthy tissues like muscles, nerves, bones, and tendons instead of fat.

How I Do Things Now

Today, with all my clients, I have them keep a food journal for at least a week. I want to not only see what they are eating and how many calories are in these foods, but we also look for areas of their diet high in carbs or pro-inflammatory vegetable oils.

Mostly, we do the food journal to help the clients bring awareness to the food they are eating. Then we have a conversation about how this food is communicating with their body.

We then set out on a journey to learn how to speak our body's love language, the language of anti-inflammatory foods. Bonjour belle!

Calories And Feelings Of Guilt

Obsessive calorie counting can also lead to feelings of guilt and shame surrounding our food.

---

[5] "Deep Nutrition: Why Your Genes Need Traditional Food: Catherine ...." https://www.amazon.com/Deep-Nutrition-Your-Genes-Traditional/dp/1250113822. Accessed 27 Sep. 2018.

When a banana is 100 calories, a slice of pizza 400 calories, and a chicken breast 300, we lose sight of the big picture. We start to think of food as simply a mathematical formula and weight loss as an inevitable byproduct of our restriction.

We start to view an hour bike ride not as a joyous time out in nature communicating well with our body but instead view it as 600 more calories to eat for the day.

Master each of the habits in this book. Learn how to create a healthy environment rich with nutritional and movement communication. The weight and health outcomes you are seeking will take care of themselves.

CHAPTER 3: REDUCE CARBS
TO UNDER 100 GRAMS

If food is a language, why would we give a specific number of grams of carbs to eat per day?

We recommend reducing carbs under 100 grams a day for two reasons. First, it's easy to remember and easy to know whether or not you've done it. Second, by keeping your carbohydrate intake low, you'll naturally eat foods that communicate well with your body.

Here are some facts about sugar:

- Our stores are full of sugary foods, making it seem like buying sugary things is the norm.
- Sugar can change our DNA and make us age more rapidly.[6]
- Sugar disrupts hormonal function.[7]
- Sugar is sticky, and when in high levels in our blood, it wreaks havoc.[8]
- There are far too many people in our world addicted to sugar. The average American consumes 220 pounds per year.[9]

---

[6] "Sugared Soda Consumption, Cell Aging Associated in New Study ...." 16 Oct. 2014, https://www.ucsf.edu/news/2014/10/119431/sugared-soda-consumption-cell-aging-associated-new-study. Accessed 25 Sep. 2018.

[7] "Your Blood Sugar May Be the Key to Your Hormone Imbalance ...." 11 Nov. 2015, https://health.clevelandclinic.org/polycystic-ovary-syndrome-pill-not-remedy/. Accessed 25 Sep. 2018.

[8] "Nutrition and aging skin: sugar and glycation. - NCBI." https://www.ncbi.nlm.nih.gov/pubmed/20620757. Accessed 25 Sep. 2018.

- A diet high in sugar changes the biochemistry of our brains to crave more sugar. It's a vicious cycle.[10]
- Sadly, carbohydrates, complex and simple, turn into sugar in our body.

As a general rule, I encourage people to keep dietary carbohydrate intake to 100 grams per day or less. 100 grams is not a hard rule backed by science. It's just a simple number that is easy to remember.

For the average person eating 2000 calories a day, this would be roughly 20% of their total calories, or 400 calories of carbohydrates.

You can track your daily sugar intake on MyFitnessPal, a free calorie-counting app, or with a pen and paper.

Do We Need Sugar To Live?

You need glucose in your bloodstream to survive. But our bodies were designed to create glucose from just about everything we eat. We start to have problems when we get too much sugar in our bloodstream. Hence the 100 grams rule.

Sugar is sparse in nature. Now we Americans consume 200-plus pounds each year!

Sugar Is Addictive

Sugar consumption releases endogenous opiates,[11] brain chemicals that make you feel so good that you do things you know are stupid just to get that feeling again. Something stupid like driving 60 minutes in LA traffic just to get some Salt & Straw ice cream like I've done. But that stuff is so good!

---

[9] "How Much Sugar Are Americans Eating? [Infographic] - Forbes." 30 Aug. 2012, https://www.forbes.com/sites/alicegwalton/2012/08/30/how-much-sugar-are-americans-eating-infographic/. Accessed 25 Sep. 2018.
[10] "This Is What Sugar Does To Your Brain | HuffPost." 6 Apr. 2015, https://www.huffingtonpost.com/2015/04/06/sugar-brain-mental-health_n_6904778.html. Accessed 25 Sep. 2018.
[11] "The relationship between opioid and sugar intake: Review of evidence ...." https://www.ncbi.nlm.nih.gov/pmc/articles/PMC3109725/. Accessed 25 Sep. 2018.

The side effects of sugar consumption include, but are not limited to, reduced immune function,[12] increased fat production,[13] fatty liver,[14] hypertension,[15] anxiety,[16] and diabetes.

Add vegetable oil to your sugary diet and these unhealthy side effects are magnified.

Here's a quick test to know if you're addicted: Does eating something sugary give you the "OMG, this is the greatest thing ever, take this from me and I will hurt you!" feeling? If so, you're addicted.

Sugar And Hormones

The average American today is 15 to 16 pounds heavier than in the 1980s.[17]

Not only are people gaining weight through life, but we are also gaining weight faster than we did a few decades ago.

This may be a result of sugar's disruptive effect on the hormones inside our body.

Like the natural and good foods we are calling you to eat, sugar also communicates with our bodies. In excess, it binds to hormone receptors and makes them insensitive to insulin.[18] Sugar blocks

---

[12] "Does Sugar Really Suppress the Immune System? - Scientific American." 21 Jul. 2018, https://www.scientificamerican.com/article/does-sugar-really-suppress-the-immune-system/. Accessed 25 Sep. 2018.

[13] "Research Links Sugar Consumption, Fat Production, and Diabetes ...." 3 Apr. 2011, http://www.yalescientific.org/2011/04/research-links-sugar-consumption-fat-production-and-diabetes/. Accessed 25 Sep. 2018.

[14] "Carbohydrate intake and nonalcoholic fatty liver disease: fructose as a ...." https://www.ncbi.nlm.nih.gov/pmc/articles/PMC4405421/. Accessed 25 Sep. 2018.

[15] "Salt and sugar: their effects on blood pressure. - NCBI." https://www.ncbi.nlm.nih.gov/pubmed/25547872. Accessed 25 Sep. 2018.

[16] "4 Ways Sugar Could Be Harming Your Mental Health | Psychology ...." https://www.psychologytoday.com/us/blog/where-science-meets-the-steps/201309/4-ways-sugar-could-be-harming-your-mental-health. Accessed 25 Sep. 2018.

[17] "Average American 15 Pounds Heavier Than 20 Years Ago." 3 Aug. 2016, https://consumer.healthday.com/public-health-information-30/centers-for-disease-control-news-120/average-american-15-pounds-heavier-than-20-years-ago-713484.html. Accessed 26 Sep. 2018.

[18] "Insulin and Insulin Resistance - NCBI - NIH." https://www.ncbi.nlm.nih.gov/pmc/articles/PMC1204764/. Accessed 26 Sep.

nutrient channels, weakens bones, and makes it more difficult to build lean tissues like muscle.[19]

For women frustrated with midlife weight gain and difficulty losing weight, sugar is often the culprit.

Sugar consumption + menopausal hormone changes = weight gain.

Sugar even changes the collagen in our joints, skin, and tendons, which can lead to early aging, arthritis, and other inflammatory issues. It also disrupts our white blood cell function, a prime protector from diseases like cancer and infections.[20]

How does sugar do all this terrible stuff?

Sugar Sticks To You

My aunt taught my sister and me how to make "taffy" as kids. Much to the dismay of our mom, we would squash and compress marshmallows until they became a gooey mess. After eating the "taffy," there would always be residue on our hands until they were thoroughly washed.

Sugar has a sticky feeling once it dissolves in water. It reacts with proteins on our skin to form breakable chemical bonds. When you pull your fingers apart, you are feeling the tug of the bonds being broken. This is the same process that occurs inside our body when there is too much sugar in our bloodstream. This is called glycation.

These reactions are temporary. But with enough time and heat, these bonds can become permanent. These reactions are called Advanced Glycation End Products (AGEs). These types of reactions do make us age rapidly.

AGEs create a stiffening of our tissues when our blood sugar level is chronically elevated.

This process can lead to atherosclerotic plaque development, joint pain, and even cancer growth.[21]

2018.

[19] "Deep Nutrition: Why Your Genes Need Traditional Food: Catherine ...." https://www.amazon.com/Deep-Nutrition-Your-Genes-Traditional/dp/1250113822. Accessed 26 Sep. 2018.

[20] "Why Sugar Is Just As Bad For Your Skin As It Is For Your Waistline ...." 10 Oct. 2013, https://www.huffingtonpost.com/2013/10/10/sugar-bad-for-skin_n_4071548.html. Accessed 26 Sep. 2018.

[21] "Deep Nutrition: Why Your Genes Need Traditional Food: Catherine ...." https://www.amazon.com/Deep-Nutrition-Your-Genes-

This is why it's so important to eat a low-carb and especially low-sugar diet.

What About Blood Vessels?

Inside our blood vessels there is a complicated series of interactions taking place thousands of times per second. Just watch the episode of "The Magic School Bus" on the human body and you'll see what I'm talking about.

It's not simply a hollow tube where blood flows through. Rather it's a complex interaction of hormones, nutrients, and blood vessels all happening at lightspeed. When glycation reactions occur and AGEs form, the flow of blood slows and there is confusion in the blood cells.

When there is confusion in our blood cells, it affects our muscles' ability to contract, our eyes' ability to process visual information, and our skin's ability to feel and sense where we are in space.

Normally, when there are issues with our circulatory system, our white blood cells come to the rescue and patch things up. But when AGEs take place, our white blood cells lose their ability to help. A loss of white blood cell function can lead to early cancer cell growth. AGEs are even the primary reason diabetics develop circulatory problems.

Certain cells require a steady supply of glucose. It's the sole job of the pancreas to make sure our blood stream has the right amount at all times. Our pancreas is highly skilled at its job.

When we eat a big piece of cake or drink a large soda, AGEs form in our blood stream. If the clean-up crew does not have enough time to clean things up before your next treat, problems start to occur as AGEs become permanent.

This is the downward spiral into which so many diabetics fall. And this is why keeping our sugar and carbohydrate intake low is so important.

Sugar And Complexity

Traditional/dp/1250113822. Accessed 26 Sep. 2018.

When we eat a free-range chicken breast cooked on the bone that we purchased from the local farmers market, we can be assured we will receive a large and complex amount of nutritional information. The chicken roamed outside, eating grass and insects and soaking up vitamin D. Juxtapose this with processed carbohydrates like granola. The granola was made in a factory and likely has artificial vitamins and minerals injected into it. We need to understand that this type of nutritional communication is different inside our bodies.

As our world's resources continue to shrink, sugar-laden foods will dominate more and more.

What Does It Look Like To Have A Carb-Conscious Day?

I've gotten quite a few questions about what a "carb-conscious" day would look like.

Well, here it is.

First, we have a sample menu with estimates for how many grams of carbs are included.

Notice the example foods. They are all low in carbs. The chili with sweet potato was the bulk of the carbs for the day.

Breakfast
- Vital Farms Free-Range Eggs: *2 grams*
- Kerrygold Grass-Fed Butter: *0 grams*
- Organic Spinach: *7 grams*

Lunch
- Homemade grass-fed ground beef chili with organic sweet potatoes: *40 grams*

Dinner
- Large organic kale salad with goat cheese, pine nuts, and homemade olive oil and vinegar dressing: *20 grams of carbs*

The total carbohydrate intake for the day was about 60 grams.

As you'll notice, when you think of food as a language that communicates with your body, it's easy to stay under the 100 grams of carbs per day. When you fill your body with nutrient-dense vegetables, fresh dairy products, and meat off the bone, it leaves little room for carbs.

What About Artificial Sweeteners?

Artificial sweeteners like Splenda and even stevia communicate something with your body that is confusing. When you ingest something sweet, your body prepares itself for a rush of glucose. It releases insulin. When there is no sugar for insulin to manage, LDL levels tend to rise and body fat is stored more readily.

I advise against the use of artificial sweeteners, even natural ones like stevia. When your body doesn't get the sugar it thinks it will get, hunger signals rise and you're more likely to overeat later on.

Focus instead on eating real foods that will communicate well with your body.

For a specific list of grams of carbs in common foods, see this website:

https://open.umich.edu/sites/default/files/downloads/diabetes_10 1-taking_charge.pdf.

George

George was an avid triathlete when he started working with our team at Village. He told me he was about 50 pounds overweight, pre-diabetic, and knew he needed to get his diet under control.

I started having him keep a food journal, and we found that most of his calories were coming from sugars in the form of fruit, premade sports products, and bread.

We set a cap at 100 grams and he obliged. Over the next few months, the weight finally started falling off. He was ecstatic!

Should I Avoid Sugar Altogether?

We've talked about the effects of sugar on our brain, skin, circulatory system, and body fat. My hope is not that you will never have ice cream or enjoy a dessert ever again. My hope is that these things will be the exception and not the norm.

My hope is that you'll make healthy fats, vegetables, and protein the main event of your meals instead of carbs.

Don't view sugary foods as "off-limits." This tends to create unhealthy psychological issues. Instead, view these foods as a poor means of nutritional communication with your body. Create a diet rich in foods that communicate well like the ones we will cover in the next chapters.

It's easy to overeat carbs. Enzymes in our mouth convert starch to sugar and increase our appetite. In your stomach, carbs tend to take up little space so we don't get full quickly, causing us to eat more than we need.

Don't ditch carbs — just rethink the ratios.

You can have the pasta, but switch out most of the noodles and add in extra sauce. Better yet, try zucchini noodles!

Have bread, but eat it slowly and with a generous helping of butter.

If you like stir-fry, heap on the meat and veggies and keep rice to a minimum.

CHAPTER 4: NATURAL FATS WON'T MAKE YOU FAT

How We Developed An Unhealthy Fear Of Fat

"I just can't wrap my head around buying full-fat products. The idea of eating full-fat cheese and real butter, and egg-yolks… I mean, that fat can't be good for me, right?" Linda said to me across the table in my office. Linda was a client of ours who was struggling to lose weight. She had cut calories and was purchasing seemingly healthy products like Lean Cuisine and Activa Low-Fat yogurt.

"My doctor says I need to watch my cholesterol, and I know full-fat products raise cholesterol," she added.

As I went on to explain to Linda, there is little reason to fear cholesterol.

I never want to come across as contradicting someone's doctor or telling them not to take medication. That's not my place. My place is simply to educate and equip our clients to be informed health consumers.

Sadly, most of modern medicine is 30 years behind in their understanding of what actually causes heart attacks.

By the end of this chapter, my hope is to educate you that natural fats like animal fats, healthy oils, and nuts are healthy, and processed fats like vegetable oil are toxic.

Toxic Fats

The fat we need to have a fear of is vegetable oil. Vegetable oil, touted for its heart-health benefits, disrupts basic cellular function, interrupts the cholesterol communication system, and creates inflammation in our body.

During processing, vegetable oils are heated and their polyunsaturated fatty acids undergo oxidative damage. What develops are mega trans fats. These mega trans fats cause inflammation, cellular breakdown, and all-out confusion inside our body.

Vegetable oil creates an environment of chaos inside us.

If you eat a steady diet of vegetable oil, it's a guarantee that it will have a negative effect on your health.

Dr. Spiteller, a lipid scientist (these people study fat for a living!), has proven through his research that oxidation of certain fats causes plaque to develop in our arteries. He says that processed polyunsaturated fats are the real culprit for the stiffening of arteries in our bodies.[22] PUFA fats are ubiquitous in vegetable oil.

Nature Can't Make Bad Fats

Some of the healthiest cultures in our world today live on a diet that is mainly fat. Yet some of the most unhealthy cultures like ours are becoming sick because of the type of fat we are eating.

The difference is that we are eating processed, vegetable oil-heavy, polyunsaturated fatty acid-laden foods. The people in the healthiest parts of the world are eating natural fats.

"Eat Natural Fats And Avoid Processed Ones" - Dr. Catherine Shanahan

Better Fat Burn

When we eat a diet full of processed low-fat foods and sugar, our fat-burning enzymes become dormant. When we reintroduce foods rich in natural fat, we reignite the fat-burning enzymes we were designed to use and make burning body fat easier. Sugar and carbs, on the other hand, make this process difficult.

---

[22] "The Cholesterol Myth." http://2fhjuw36qc3g36anx54adxd2nje.wpengine.netdna-cdn.com/wp-content/uploads/2011/07/CholMythCamb1.pdf. Accessed 26 Sep. 2018.

Less Junk Food

When our metabolism is full of nutrients and fullness-inducing healthy fats, we will be less hungry. But when we are filled with processed foods and aren't given the full-fat communication our body craves, we will look outside the body to fill the void. This means filling up on sugar, starch, and fake vegetable oil-laden fats. These things may taste good, but the taste comes through artificial means.

Essential Nutrients

Natural fats are an integral part of an optimal diet. You can live without them, but you won't thrive. Our body needs natural fats to break down, digest, and absorb the nutrients from the vegetables we will talk about in the next chapter.

Prevent Nutrient Loss During Cooking

Natural fats protect our food during the cooking process. They keep meat moist, preserve nutrients, and create an environment for health. Cook meat less to preserve essential nutrients and make your food as healthy as possible.

The Conspiracy Of Cholesterol

In the 1950s a man named Ancel Keys starred in a CBS documentary called "The Search." On the show, Keys claimed to have found the cause for heart disease.

He used bad statistics to peg the rise in heart attacks on natural fats. His research was used by margarine manufacturers to make it seem like margarine was a healthy alternative to saturated fat-laden butter. The world's producers of margarine were ecstatic as sales began to skyrocket.

Unfortunately we got the story all wrong. Ancel Keys claimed fat was clogging our arteries like a clogged pipe. His analogy was false and led to decades of poor nutritional communication.

So, should we believe Ancel Keys, who did his PhD on electric eels, or hundreds of lipid scientists who study fat for a living?

Lipid scientists have been arguing for decades that natural fats and cholesterol have always been part of the human diet and are not the problem.

Sadly, heart attacks have steadily risen to become the number-one killer of Americans as vegetable oil consumption has increased and butter and other animal fat consumption decreased.

The real problem lies in polyunsaturated fatty acids. At Village, we refer to them as PUFAs. It's easy to remember because they make our arteries go "poof!" These are chemically unstable molecules and they are abundant in vegetable oil.

In 2001, nutrition scientists at the Harvard School of Public Health went on to suggest that the low-fat, anti-cholesterol theory of health was not only dead wrong, but it was setting people up to be more likely to have diabetes and heart disease.[23]

As more research is discovering that animal fats are healthy, the pressure is building towards change in medicine. However, the medical guidelines remain the same, and thus you won't likely hear this from your primary care physician.

So how did Ancel Keys convince America that animal fats were bad?

He used bad science. Keys did not compare PUFA fats to animal fats. Instead he compared PUFAs to artificial trans fats (a toxic fat).

He claimed to have tested saturated fats when in reality he was testing trans fat-laden vegetable oils. How he made the connection between these vegetable oils and animal products, we are not sure.

Trans fats have been proven to raise cholesterol. Foods containing artificially made saturated fat, like margarine and shortenings, contain plenty of trans fat. These foods have been clearly shown to elevate cholesterol when added to a diet that was previously free of these foods.

This was enough to convince modern medicine, however, and natural fats have been taboo ever since.

The Data Ancel Keys Neglected To Publish

---

[23] "Eggs | The Nutrition Source | Harvard T.H. Chan School of Public Health." https://www.hsph.harvard.edu/nutritionsource/food-features/eggs/. Accessed 26 Sep. 2018.

Medical detective work by Christopher E. Ramsden, medical investigator at the NIH, who published an article called "Re-evaluation of the traditional diet-heart hypothesis: analysis of recovered data from Minnesota Coronary Experiment (1968-73)",[24] implicates Keys in one of the greatest nutrition scandals of the age.

Both groups in Keys' study were at an increased risk of heart attack. We know that trans fats increase risk for heart attack. But according to even Ancel Keys' data, so do PUFA fats.

A Nurses Health Study showed that for each 2% increase in trans fat in the diet, the risk of heart disease is doubled.[25] What's crazy is that the trans-fat diet performed *better* than the PUFA diet. **This suggests that vegetable oil has a more toxic impact on our health than even trans fats.**

In spite of progress in the realm of saturated fat, doctors still have a long way to go in understanding the health consequences of consuming polyunsaturated fats from industrially produced vegetable oils. Nutrition science as a whole has made very little progress on this front in large part because Ancel Keys appears to have done everything in his power to keep us from understanding just how unhealthy PUFAs and vegetable oils are.

Keys misled people to believe that saturated fats, like those found in eggs and butter, were to blame for the atherosclerotic plaques in our body. However, the polyunsaturated fats in the hydrogenated oils he used in his experiments were the real culprit.

Thanks to great books like *Deep Nutrition* and *The Primal Blueprint*, Americans have come a long way in their understanding of how trans fats are the actual problem and how saturated fats from natural sources are healthy and communicate well with our bodies. Even a handful of doctors today are starting to lift the restrictions on eggs and butter to allow folks to enjoy these amazingly healthy foods! But until the medical guidelines are changed to match current research, you won't likely see many doctors going against the herd mentality and changing what they recommend.

---

[24] "Re-evaluation of the traditional diet-heart hypothesis: analysis of ...." 12 Apr. 2016, https://www.bmj.com/content/353/bmj.i1246. Accessed 26 Sep. 2018.
[25] "Trans fatty acids – A risk factor for cardiovascular disease - NCBI - NIH." https://www.ncbi.nlm.nih.gov/pmc/articles/PMC3955571/. Accessed 26 Sep. 2018.

Best Sources Of Healthy Fat
- Free-range, grass-fed, organic, on-the-bone meat
- Full-fat, pasture-raised dairy
- Whole, raw milk
- Eggs from free-range chickens
- Nuts and seeds
- Avocados
- Salmon and other fatty fish
- Coconut and coconut oil
- The oils mentioned above

Can I Eat Meat?

Have you been watching the Netflix documentaries lately about the dangers of meat consumption?

If so, you've likely developed a fear of animal products.

I remember the day after I watched the documentary *What The Health*. I remember eating a piece of organic grass-fed chicken that my wife prepared and thinking, "Is this wrecking my arteries and causing cancer?"

I've had numerous friends tell me how great they feel after switching to a vegetarian or vegan diet. But I don't think we can assume just because someone feels good when they switch to a vegan diet that the reason they feel good is a reduction in meat consumption.

We also need to consider the drastic drop-off in processed foods in the vegetarian life.

Reduced consumption or elimination of poorly sourced meats from feedlots is probably the real reason why people feel good.

I've also heard stories of folks who've gone vegan and then added back in grass-fed beef, organic free-range chicken breast and still felt amazing.

I think the problem with meat consumption is not meat consumption itself. The real problem is the toxic and harmful conditions the meat is raised under and the effect that has on how this food communicates with our body.

As I learn more about the anti-inflammatory diet and the way we as humans were intended to eat, I've come to believe that not all meat consumption is equal.

The food we eat communicates with our body. When you put chicken into your system that has been raised inhumanely in a crowded environment while being pumped full of antibiotics and other chemicals, you are communicating that environment to your body.

On the other hand, when you eat a chicken with the meat cooked on the bone from an organic, free-range chicken, it creates a whole different language of communication. The microecology of the chicken gets transferred to your body, communicating wellness.

There are numerous benefits to allowing the cow, chicken, buffalo, or whatever other meat you eat to forage in the grass and live in an open and healthy environment. The animals, when in a natural living condition, are going to be much healthier. In turn, when you consume them, that health will be transferred to you.

Meats With Bone And Skin Are Better Than Boneless And Skinless

When I first started in the fitness industry, I thought the epitome of health was boneless, skinless chicken breast with steamed broccoli atop brown rice.

Whenever I had a meal like this, I always had to suffer through it one dry, miserable bite at a time. "I'm willing to do what it takes to be healthy," I told myself.

Thankfully I was wrong.

Healthy food is supposed to be flavorful *naturally*.

"Well, what about fast food?" you ask. "I think fast food tastes good."

Yes, fast food does taste good. But this is simply because fast food companies like McDonald's and Taco Bell use artificial flavoring agents like MSG, sugar, and free glutamate to enhance flavor.

When we think of health food as bland, flavorless chicken, it's difficult to compete with fast food.

But when we think of health food as savory meat with the bone still in and the fat and skin still on, it will open up a wide and rich world of flavor.

29

When we cook meat with bones still in, the minerals and nutrients from the bone are absorbed into the meats, which in turn are transferred to our body to help keep our joints and tissues healthy. When we eat meat that still has the skin on, it preserves the natural fats, helping to make us better fat burners and improving the health of our joints by increasing the amount of collagen in our system.

Most importantly, meat on the bone with the skin on tastes better, making us more likely to continue eating an amazingly healthy food.

Can I Eat Too Much Fat?

Yes.

But for most people, the problem is not that they get too many calories (though they often do); it's that they get too few nutrients, and their body is telling them to eat more than they should.

Instead of focusing on eating fewer calories, think about eating more nutrients.

It goes without saying that if your desire is to eat as many nutrient-dense foods as you can in favor of those foods that lack nutritional power, you'll necessarily be eating fewer empty calories — and that's the point.

Listen to your body. It is craving nutrient-dense foods. So eat them in abundance and create an environment of health.

CHAPTER 5: YES, YOU NEED TO EAT LOTS OF VEGGIES

Michael Pollan, of nutrition-world fame, said the following: "Eat real food. Not too much. Mostly plants."

I think vegetable consumption is the only nutritional recommendation I've never heard anyone contradict. In fact, eating more vegetables, and a wide variety of vegetables, is the most well-respected and often-given nutritional advice.

When I sit down with clients, they nearly always tell me that they eat healthy. But "healthy" means different things for different people. For some people, eating healthy means having the oatmeal with a heart symbol on the container, raisins, and brown sugar with skim milk for breakfast. For others, it means having vegetables at dinner.

Nearly everyone we coach needs to eat more vegetables.

We recommend five servings a day, minimum.

A serving of vegetables is about one fistful (more on this soon).

Vegetable consumption is difficult in our society today. We live in a world that seeks instant gratification, fast food, and leaves little time for cooking a nutritious meal.

Adding three to five servings of vegetables to your life is going to be difficult if you don't do it already.

If you decide to eat a wide variety of vegetables and choose organic like we suggest below, your grocery bill will likely go up. You also need to spend more time learning how to prepare veggie-dense meals.

I'll go as far as to say that the increased cost of time and money required to add more vegetables to your life is a good thing. Your credit card statement is a good indicator of your priorities. If you're spending more on your food and your fitness, you'll value your body more. You'll see your health as an investment, and your body is something you want to nourish and care for.

In this chapter, I'm going to try to make vegetable consumption as cost-effective and efficient as possible.

"Why use fists?" your inquisitive mind might be thinking. Well, not everyone has scales or measuring cups with them all the time, but most of us have hands with us at all times.

Simply make your hand into a fist and you have the size of one serving of vegetables.

Now, get five of them in throughout the day.

Vegetable Basics

Not all vegetables are created equal. In this next section, we will talk about the differences between starchy and non-starchy vegetables and which veggies you should bias yourself towards.

Non-Starchy Vegetables

Characteristics of non-starchy vegetables are:
- Low in calories
- Low in carbohydrates
- Low in sugar
- High in water
- High in fiber
- High in nutrients

These are all great. When we talk about communicating well with our body, we should think of adding a wide nutritional bandwidth and a plethora of nutrients. Vegetables, because they're relatively low in calories and carbohydrates, are not going to fill us very quickly, but they're loaded with nutrients, fiber, and communicate amazingly with our body. This is especially true for non-starchy vegetables.

Let me go as far as to say that having a serving of non-starchy vegetables at every single meal could be the one habit you need in your life to lose weight, be healthy, and have the body you want.

Examples Of Non-Starchy Vegetables:
- All "Leafy Greens" (Spinach, Kale, Romaine, etc.)
- Asparagus
- Broccoli
- Brussels Sprouts
- Celery
- Cabbage (all kinds)
- Carrots
- Cauliflower
- Cucumbers
- Mushrooms
- Onions (Yellow, Red)
- Peppers (Red, Orange, Yellow, Green)
- Sprouts
- Tomatoes
- Yellow Squash
- Zucchini

Feel free to eat as many of these non-starchy veggies as you would like. Because they're so low in calories and so high in nutrients, you really can't overdo it.

Starchy Vegetables
- Higher in calories
- Higher in carbs and starches
- Higher in sugar
- Moderately high in nutrients
- High in water content

Starchy vegetables, on the other hand, need to be eaten in moderation. Although I would certainly not put these in the category of a "bad" food, they are loaded with carbohydrates and thus should be in moderation to keep total carbohydrate count low.

Examples Of Starchy Vegetables:
- Squash (Butternut, Acorn, Spaghetti)
- Pumpkin
- Beets
- Potatoes and Sweet Potatoes
- Turnips
- Rutabaga
- Peas
- Corn (not actually a vegetable but a grain, yet most people count it as a vegetable, so that's why it's listed here)

How Much Should I Eat?

You want to aim for five "fists" of vegetables per day. Ideally, the majority of those fists would come from non-starchy vegetables. Strive for three to five fists of non-starchy vegetables and two fists or less of starchy vegetables. As long as you're keeping your carbohydrate intake under 100 grams a day, feel free to include starchy veggies.

How To Make Veggies Taste Good

"With Enough Butter, Anything Is Good" - Julia Child

When eaten without butter or salt, veggies are often bland, unappetizing, and a chore to consume.

As we learned in the previous chapter, the myths surrounding saturated fat consumption are downright wrong.

One of my goals as a nutrition coach is to get people to actually enjoy eating vegetables. I think you can force yourself to eat three to five servings of veggies for a while. The especially disciplined person may be able to do it for a long time. But why suffer needlessly?

Here's permission to add butter, coconut oil, bacon grease, and salt to your vegetables.

Not only will this make weight loss easier, but your risk for heart attack, Alzheimer's, and even diabetes will decrease.

I would even say that vegetables not only taste better but are *healthier* when we add fat and salt to them.

Most of the veggies' flavorful parts are locked behind a wall of cellulose (the strong outer part of the veggies). Our saliva and teeth can't break down these walls.

Fat also ensures nutrient absorption in our bloodstream.

Try dipping carrots, bell peppers, and/or celery in a yogurt-dill dressing. Butter, sauces, dressings, dips, and spreads are your key to ensuring you get five servings of veggies each day and actually like it.

Eat The Rainbow

We're not talking about Skittles here. We're talking vegetables!

Strive to eat as many different colors of vegetables throughout your day as possible. See the different color as an array of different parts of healthy communication with your body.

Color is important because it represents nutrient, vitamin, and antioxidant variety. Having a wide nutrient bandwidth is essential to having a healthy diet.

Nature's way of letting us know a food is full of antioxidants and good nutritional communication is though color.

These colors indicate nutrient content and also the presence of antioxidants, phytochemicals, and other free radical-fighting ninjas that are important in slowing down the aging process and helping our body deal with inflammation. This is especially important in our world of sugar and vegetable oil consumption.

When clients drop their carbohydrate intake, they tend to lose weight fairly quickly. Sometimes, however, they hit a plateau, and weight loss stalls. The way to avoid hitting a plateau and continue losing weight until you hit your ideal is to have a wide bandwidth of nutritional communication with your body.

This means eating a variety of different vegetables. Don't just eat spinach salads for lunch every day and think you've checked the veggie box. Try to branch out and have a kale salad or some other type of lettuce.

Eat More Vegetables Than Fruits

Before modern farming, fruit was difficult to come by and only eaten in season. Today, thanks to GMOs, we can have most fruits year-round and as often as we want.

35

Vegetables have much less sugar and calories than fruits. Even though sugar in fruit is "natural" sugar, it is still sugar nonetheless.

Now, would we rather have you eat fruit than a bowl of ice cream? You bet.

Fruits are loaded with antioxidants, vitamins, fiber, water, and phytonutrients. Phytonutrients protect us from illness and help make us healthier.

We recommend eating three servings of vegetables for every serving of fruit.

The reason is because fruit has a lot of sugar in it. Excessive sugar consumption — even good sugar — can promote weight gain, make losing weight tougher, and contribute to the inflammatory process.

If you're trying to keep your carbs under 100 grams each day, having just one banana brings your daily carb total to 27 grams.

Most people with no specific health conditions (like diabetes, for example) who are moderately active can eat between one to two servings of fruit a day without a problem; those who exercise a lot can get by with a little more.

The type of fruit you have matters a lot in terms of the nutrients and sugar content that you get. But even more importantly: Eat whole, real fruit.

It's a good idea to eat a range of whole pieces of fruits to make sure you get the full spectrum of benefits that different fruits offer.

Check out some of the health benefit highlights of different popular fruits:

- Blueberries are high in antioxidants, fiber, Vitamin C, manganese.
- Strawberries are relatively low in sugar, low in calories, high in Vitamin C, high in anti-inflammatory plant-phenols.
- Grapefruit is high in vitamin A, B6, and C, high in fiber, potassium, pantothenic acid, thiamine, magnesium, and copper, rich in antioxidants.
- Bananas are high in vitamins C and B6, high in fiber, potassium, and manganese, a good source of folate, magnesium and copper, rich in antioxidants.

I think it's great to eat fruit. Just use moderation.

Make A Giant Bowl Of Salad

Nicole and I use our giant, silver mixing bowls to make our salads each time we eat them.

Start by loading up with a mix of different greens. We use kale, spinach, swiss chard, and micro greens. Then pack on the toppings. Nuts and seeds, fermented veggies, endive, or anything else.

I always add cheese to give it some creaminess. Our family favorite is goat cheese.

Now that you've made this amazing salad, don't wreck it by topping it with vegetable oil dressing. Make your own simple dressing with olive oil and balsamic vinegar.

Stir Fry And Steam

These are the other two easiest ways to get veggies in. I love a good sauteed onion and bell pepper with my eggs in the morning.

You also can't go wrong with steamed broccoli topped with goat cheese, sesame seeds, and raisins.

Fermented Vegetables

Neither Nicole nor I grew up eating anything fermented (dill pickles from Mrs. Vick's don't count).

We were both pretty skeptical when we started our journey with fermented food. After reading about the health wonders of fermented foods, we both journeyed to Sprouts and headed to the back left corner where there was an open refrigerator section of unique health foods. We proceeded to grab a bag of fermented carrots, pickles, sauerkraut, and kimchi. Within the next week we tried all of them and even gave our son, Cooper, some too. He didn't like any of them, and Nicole and I took a while to develop an affinity towards them.

But after some time, we found recipes using different fermented foods that taste really great.

Today, we eat Bubbies pickles for snacks, make a salad with sauerkraut, and I often have kimchi atop my eggs.

Why Fermented Foods?

The bacteria in fermented foods are capable of transforming bland, tasteless, and even toxic compounds into edible and healthy wonders.

Fermented foods add complexity to the bacterial community in our gut that helps us to fight off bacteria and bolsters our immune system.

Here are three of my favorite veggie recipes:

Massaged Kale Salad:

Ingredients:
- 2 bunches of organic Lacinato Kale
- Drizzle of olive oil
- 1-2 Tbsp of apple cider vinegar
- Juice of 1 large lemon
- 1 can of garbanzo beans
- 1 carrot, shredded
- 1 large or 2 small avocados, cubed
- 1 small container of goat cheese or feta cheese
- ¼ cup of sauerkraut

Directions:

1. The key to this recipe is massaging the kale. First cut up the kale into small pieces and remove the large part of the stems (they are hard to chew).

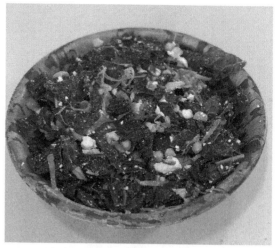

2. Place the kale in a big bowl and run water over it until it fills to the top. Let the kale sit there for a couple of minutes to make sure all the dirt and sediment drop to the bottom of the bowl. Carefully grab the kale from the top of the bowl and place it into a salad spinner. Then spin the kale until it is fairly dry.

3. Once the kale is dryish, place in a large bowl and drizzle with a generous amount of olive oil, apple cider vinegar, and lemon juice. This is the fun part... Now go to work and massage all of the juices into the kale until it has the kale down into the bowl by at least a quarter of the way and all of the kale leaves are covered in the marinade. Then cover the bowl and stick in the fridge to marinade for at least a few hours, but preferably overnight.

4. Remove the kale from the fridge and top with all the other delicious toppings and toss. Enjoy!

Caramelized Onions

Ingredients:
-   White or yellow onions (in my recipe, I used 2 large sweet yellow onions)
-   Generous amount of avocado oil
-   Salt
-   Grass-fed butter

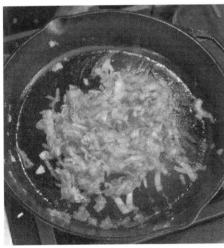

Directions:
1. Heat cast-iron skillet on low-medium with avocado oil.
2. Cut onions into long, thin slices.
3. Place onion slices into cast-iron skillet and stir until they are broken up. Then cover with a lid. Check on onions every 3-5 minutes and stir intermittently.
4. Once the onions have reduced down, add a bit of grass-fed butter and salt.
5. Stir the onions until they are soft and light brown. If they start to get really dark, reduce heat so they don't blacken.
6. Enjoy the onions on top of anything — eggs, salad, meat — they add a lot of flavor!

Chicken Veggie Stir-Fry

Ingredients:

- Bone-in organic chicken breasts (1-2 depending on how many people you are feeding)
- Avocado oil or ghee
- Salt
- Pepper
- Coconut oil
- 1 green bell pepper, cut into long, thin slices
- 1 red bell pepper, cut into long, thin slices
- 1 bunch of broccoli, cut into bite-size pieces
- 1 medium onion, cut into long, thin slices
- 3-4 medium carrots, diced into thin, bite-size pieces
- 1 zucchini, cut into long, thin slices
- 2 small lemons or 1 large lemon
- ¼ cup tahini
- 1 tsp Herbs de Provence
- Salt and Pepper to taste

Directions for chicken:

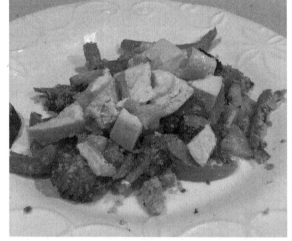

1. Coat the chicken breasts in avocado oil or ghee and sprinkle with salt and pepper.

2. Bake on a baking sheet for 15-25 minutes at 375 degrees until the chicken comes out juicy but cooked all the way through.

3. Cut chicken into bite-size pieces and place off to the side. You may save the bones to make bone broth. :)

Directions for veggie stir-fry:

1.   Heat wok or large frying pan with coconut oil on medium-high heat until it is hot.
2.   Add onions and carrots. Stir until they start to soften, about 3-5 minutes.
3.   Add the rest of the veggies: bell peppers, broccoli, zucchini. Stir until they start to soften, about 5-7 minutes.
4.   Then add lemon juice, tahini, herbs, and season with salt and pepper to taste. If you like lemon juice, add more. You may also add other seasonings you enjoy.
5.   Serve hot and top with chicken. Enjoy!

What About Juice?

Dried fruit and fruit juices are a no-no. They provide too much sugar without enough fiber and bulk. This means you consume a lot of carbs, calories, and sugar without feeling full.

They also miss the boat when it comes to communicating with your body in the way this food was meant to communicate.

Green juice, cold pressed, can be a great way to get nutrients and solid nutritional communication without having to do any cooking. However, many green drinks are still loaded with sugar and calories. The trick is to find one that's relatively low in sugar and calories. Think less than 50 calories per bottle. This lets you know that it's more vegetable than fruit.

Some green juices don't have nutritional information as they're made in-house. In this case, you need to read the ingredient labels and go by taste. If you see fruits like apples, pears, or oranges near the top of the ingredient list, it's probably sugary. Then you can go by taste. If it tastes sweet, there's probably some sugar in it.

You have to read ingredient labels. Don't become a victim to the marketing of health food companies. Pick the product up, turn it around, and question every ingredient.

What About Frozen Veggies?

We talked about the importance of nutrient density. The more nutrients food has, the better it will communicate with your body. The wider nutritional bandwidth you present your body with on a day-to-day, month-to-month, and year-to-year basis, the more fully and healthfully your genetic code will be expressed.

This is why it's so important to eat fresh vegetables instead of frozen or canned.

Fresh vegetables contain the nutrients we are intended to receive from those vegetables in their intended form for digestion. Canning damages nutrients by fusing them together, turning them into useless compounds.

When vegetables are frozen, they lose not only their flavor but also their nutrient density as well.

Feeding your kids frozen vegetables is a great way to make them veggie haters. These veggies lack flavor and often become soft and mushy when you cook them instead of crisp and crunchy.

I think in a pinch I would rather have people eat frozen vegetables than not at all, but I would definitely recommend fresh vegetables.

Fermented vegetables, which we talked about earlier, are a different story. Fermentation preserves nutrient density and adds additional bacterial friends to the mix.

How About Supplements And Powders?

Nutrients were mean to be digested in their natural form. No matter how many claims the bottle of pills makes that it's "Just Real Food" in capsule form, nothing can substitute for the real thing.

In fact, most nutraceutical companies are a complete scam and a waste of your hard-earned money.

I think this is a good time for me to go on a rant about supplements. The supplement industry is one of the most shady, corrupt, and lucrative areas of Health and Fitness.

My journey with supplements began at the age of 11, when I started drinking Slim-Fast shakes in an attempt to lose weight. It was the first time I ever "dieted," and I ended up losing about 10 pounds within a few months. But I didn't realize that the reason I lost weight wasn't because of the Slim-Fast shakes but because I ate way too much food normally and Slim-Fast shakes have barely any calories.

There is a reason the ladies who are selling protein shakes are driving Mercedes Benzes they won because of their protein powder-selling skills.

Nicole and I have been approached more times than I can count by various supplement sellers to push them on our clients. It first started when I was a personal trainer at the age of 18 and another trainer wanted me to sell a specific brand of protein powder to my clients.

At the end of the day, I really don't care what supplement you're selling. I don't care if it's cold pressed, "actually real food," organic, or made using some other fancy buzzword that is trending today.

What people actually need is to eat real food. Our bodies were designed to receive nutritional communication in the form of food.

That's why when you walk into Village today, you don't see supplements lining our shelves. If I wanted to run a more profitable business, we could sell supplements. Our clients trust us. If we told them that they needed to buy a certain brand of protein powder, a greens supplement, and to take some special probiotic pills, most of them would do it. They would be likely to buy those supplements from us and we would profit.

But I find this line of thinking contradictory with the mission and core values of our business. I want people to spend all of their money that they have set aside for their health on coaching, accountability, and real food. These are the things that will communicate well with your body.

If you are truly too busy to eat a meal and need to use a supplemental form of food to eat healthy, the first thing I would do is question your busyness. Are you a parent of an infant? Are you in a family crisis? Or is your busyness just a function of your job, kids, and everyday life? If it's the latter, I recommend you ask yourself what's truly important to you. If it's your health and being able to care for your family well a decade or two from now, I would recommend carving out some time to cook food each and every day. It will actually take less time than you think.

How To Bulk Cook Veggies

Bulk cooking veggies ahead of time is a simple trick to ensure you get your three to five servings of veggies every day of the week. Although you have great intentions of sticking to your newfound veggie habit throughout the week, by the time Wednesday hits, life has gotten crazy. Whether it's the kids' soccer practices, new assignments at work, or just the general willpower fatigue that many of us succumb to, even the best of intentions get squashed.

By bulk cooking ahead of time, you eliminate a lot of the willpower and time necessary to eat healthy throughout the week. So, set aside an hour or two on Sunday to prep for the week to set yourself up for success and to ensure you get your three to five servings of veggies.

Raw Veggies

I don't recommend buying the ready-to eat-variety of veggies for a few reasons. Usually they're not sourced well. They come from large-production farms, which care little about not using pesticides and producing a good product. Also, these pre-cut veggies tend to have less nutrients and go bad quicker. Nicole and I (actually just Nicole... let's be honest) will usually cut up celery, bell peppers, and carrots each week to have as snacks. We also dice bell peppers and onions to saute for our eggs each morning.

The process is pretty simple. First you need to buy the veggies from the store. Then once you get home, put them all in a strainer in the sink, clean, and prep. Lay them out on a cutting board and get them as close to ready-to-eat as possible. Then dry them off and package them up for the fridge.

Best Raw Veggies To Prepare in Bulk:
- Bell Peppers (red, orange, yellow, green)
- Carrots
- Grape Tomatoes
- Red Onions

Roasting Vegetables

Roasting vegetables enhances their flavor and makes them easier to digest.

Get out a flat pan and lay your veggies out across it. I recommend using avocado oil and a little bit of sea salt for a roasting. You can also add various spices to the mix to change things up. Some folks like to wait until after they roast it to add the spice, which is fine, too.

Cook at 350 to 400 degrees until vegetables are tender. Typical cooking time is 30 to 60 minutes, depending on the denseness of the veggie and the amount you cook at once.

Best Veggies to Roast:
- Asparagus
- Bell Peppers
- Broccoli
- Brussels Sprouts
- Cauliflower
- Onions (red and yellow)
- Potatoes (sweet and baby red)
- Tomatoes (large)
- Zucchini and Yellow Squash

Grilling Veggies

Simply fire up the grill and lay the veggies straight on or wrap them in tin foil. Again, I would use an oil with a high smoke point like avocado oil. Olive oil has a smoke point of about 375 degrees Fahrenheit, which is well below the normal grilling temperature.

Once on the grill, cook the veggies until they are tender.

Best Veggies to Grill:
- Asparagus
- Bell Peppers
- Eggplant
- Onions
- Mushrooms

How to Eat:
- Skewered
- Salads
- Mixed with whole grains, like quinoa

- Serve alongside protein and healthy fats

Best Veggies to Saute:
Any veggie will work well here.

This lesson is simple but extremely important. If you learn to cook in bulk each week, your likelihood of success will go up exponentially. You will always have vegetables ready to eat and add to your meals.

My Wife, Nicole
Growing up, my wife, Nicole, hated vegetables. The only vegetables she ever tried were steamed broccoli, green beans, and iceberg lettuce salads.

When she was in college, a friend asked her if she could make brussels sprouts for dinner. Nicole replied, "I really don't like brussels sprouts."

"You've never had brussels sprouts like these," her friend responded. "Just try them."

Nicole obliged. "Wow! These are actually really good."

The key was that her friend had used olive oil, salt, and other seasonings in appropriate amounts to bring out the amazing flavor in a brussels sprout.

Now Nicole is an avid vegetable eater and cooker. We nearly always have some sort of vegetable on the side of our meals at dinner every night, and we usually have sauteed spinach, kale, onions, and bell peppers in our eggs at breakfast.

CHAPTER 6: EAT TO 80% FULL

Finish What's On Your Plate

I grew up in a household where we ate fairly healthy. My mom cooked all of our meals at home and packed my lunches.

But I was still overweight. I attribute this completely to overeating. As a kid, I ate *a lot* of food.

I can't tell you how many times I've heard the story, "My parents made me finish everything on my plate when I was a kid."

There's deep-rooted psychology surrounding how we eat, how much we eat, and how food affects our bodies. Being repeatedly told as a kid that we need to finish everything on our plates, we will be more likely to overeat as adults.

Our bodies have a built-in fullness-regulation mechanism. As our stomach starts to get more full, we go through hormonal changes that create the feeling of fullness.

The problem is that these hormones take a while to kick in, so before you know it, you've continued eating well past the point of enough and progressed towards stuffed.

What Is "80% Full"?

Do you remember last Thanksgiving? Did you eat a ton of food? If so, I would consider this post-holiday, belt-busting, I'm-comfortable-pants, stuffed feeling "150% full."

"80% full" is just enough. This is the point where you don't need any more food. You just start to get the feeling of fullness in your stomach. This is why you should stop eating. Now, if this is confusing right off the bat, don't stress out. This is a high-level skill that takes practice.

To get started with this habit, simply stop eating sooner than you normally would. If you usually have three pieces of pizza in your Friday night dinner, have two.

If you eat the same foods everyday, you probably have a pretty good idea of your current portion sizes. For example, if you have oatmeal with breakfast every morning, you likely eat about the same amount each day. So tomorrow, try scooping 20% of the oatmeal out of your bowl and into Tupperware. Put it in the fridge and save it for later.

When you're out at a restaurant, save one-third of the meal for when you get home. If this is too tempting, you can simply box up part of the meal before you even start eating.

You can also try to simply leave a few bites on your plate every time you eat.

For someone who grew up in the "finish everything on your plate" world, this is a difficult exercise.

Smaller Plates

Interestingly, there is a ton of research on the psychology of small plates. When we eat with a smaller plate, we eat less.[26]

Parkinson's law states that things expand to fill the space you give them. This could apply to things like our time expanding to fill the hours we have to complete a task or our food expanding to fill out plates.

The Hunger Game

When my son, Cooper, was a newborn, one of the biggest challenges for us was keeping him awake long enough to eat. He couldn't keep his little eyes open long enough!

Eating to 80% full would be much easier if you had trouble staying awake long enough to consume everything on your plate.

---

[26] "Use Small Plates to Lose Weight | Food and Brand Lab." https://foodpsychology.cornell.edu/JACR/Small_Plates_Lose_Weight. Accessed 26 Sep. 2018.

When Cooper was hungry, he let us know by sucking on his hands or doing funny things with his lips or by crying very angrily.

Unlike a baby, many of us eat when we're not even hungry. We have lost touch with our feelings of hunger and satiety.

We eat for comfort, distraction, or routine.

So today, try asking yourself this question: Am I hungry right now?

How do you know?

Take a minute. Check in. Put your hand on your belly. What do you feel?

Do you need to eat right now? Do you want to eat right now? Do you feel like you should eat right now?

Make a game of it as you practice.

Play The Hunger Game

At every meal today:

1. Ask yourself beforehand, "Am I physically hungry?" If you don't know, that's OK. See if you can notice your own physical cues. Try to learn them. Pause for a moment and see what you notice.

2. Eat slowly.

3. Stop after each bite.

4. Check in with your body, especially your stomach sensations.

5. Ask yourself, "Am I still physically hungry?"

If yes, take another bite. Eat it mindfully. Pause again to observe your body cues.

If no, stop eating.

6. When you stop, check in with yourself. Notice what that's like, to stop. Take a moment. What thoughts come up? What sensations? Sit with that for a moment.

I call this a "game" because it's not meant to be serious. You don't need to worry about whether you're "76% full" or "83% full." Just get the general concept here.

You're playing with your hunger. Testing the edges of it. Seeing if you can sit with it for a little while. Learning your own body cues and signals. Experimenting.

Whatever comes up, just say, "Huh, that's interesting," and make a mental note of it.

My Dad

When I think of eating until 80% full, I always think of my dad. He has been nearly the exact same, lean weight since I was born. He's a normal guy, works a desk job, eats normal food, has a beer most nights, and exercises four to five times per week. But I noticed something — the dude stops eating when he's full. I've virtually never seen him have seconds of anything. And let's be honest: Are seconds really as tasty as firsts? Nope.

Now we move to me.

From an early age, I finished what was on my plate and then went after my sister's plate. I would even try to steal her breakfast sausage before I'd finished my own. She would get so mad!

I've always finished my plate. Twenty minutes later I'm often regretful, bloated, and stuffed. I've gotten better, but my natural pattern is still overeating. I don't know why. I attribute it to being overfed as a youngling.

Rate Your Hunger

This is an activity that has really helped me to quantify how hungry I am and to know when I need to eat.

Put your hunger on a scale from 1 to 10.

1 is no-desire-to-eat-whatsoever. Like *stuffed*.

10 is the hungriest you've ever been, like "my vision is going black and I would eat parsley even though I hate parsley" kind of hunger. (Seriously though, how come that stuff looks so much like cilantro and is always right next to it?)

Before each meal, pause. Ask yourself, "Am I physically hungry?" If so, how hungry?

Rank your hunger on the scale.

If you're at 7 or above, it's time to grub!

I think having just three meals a day and not snacking can help ensure you're hungry come mealtime. Also eating to 80% full will help you to be hungry for the next time you eat.

As you eat, continue to check in. When your hunger gets to a 2 or a 3, you're probably at 80% full and it's time to stop.

Again, notice what this stopping point feels like. Or what thoughts come up (e.g. "Oh no! I'm wasting food!").

I've found I justify finishing what's on my plate with irrational thoughts like "I'm not sure when I will eat again, so I should make sure I get enough now." This sort of scarcity mindset leads to overeating and makes it tough to be in tune with the natural hunger cues in our body.

Psychologically, when food was scarce thousands of years ago, eating everything you can each time you eat was important. But today, in a society where food is abundant, this is detrimental.

Things That Make Eating To 80% Difficult

Processed foods, vegetable oil, and sugar override the body's natural fullness cues and make it harder to stop when full. Alcohol also lowers inhibitions, as I'm sure you know, and makes it more likely you'll eat until stuffed.

Paul

Paul just had blood work done. His doc said it's the best it's ever been. EVERYTHING: blood sugar, LDL, HDL, his weight is down like 40 pounds. He feels better than any time he can remember.

How did he do it?

Paul made eating slowly, eating to 80% full, and working out at Village an integral part of his life. Paul didn't want to track calories or have to keep a food journal.

"I'm really busy," Paul said. "I simply don't have time to write everything down on the day that I eat."

As his brain and body got used to eating slowly, the weight started falling off, and Paul is one happy camper. More importantly, he now appreciates the food he eats more and is more conscious of the food decisions he makes.

Paul recommends setting a slow-eating timer when you're getting started with eating slowly. Be the last person at the table to start eating and finish well after everyone else!

Paul, you are the man, and we are so excited to be part of your journey!

CHAPTER 7: EAT SLOWLY AND MINDFULLY

WHY do you eat as much as you do?

If you're like most people, you think the amount you eat is driven by hunger or how much you like a given food. You probably think you're too smart to be tricked by labels, marketing, or any other psychological phenomena.

Research shows that most of us don't eat as much as we do because of hunger or how much we like a given food.[27]

We eat as much as we do and what we eat because of our environment.

The average person makes about 200 eating decisions per day.[28]

"Do I eat the piece of chocolate in my desk at work?"

"Should I finish my bagel? I'm getting full, I think."

"Do I want Chinese or Mediterranean?"

Many of these decisions are happening on a subconscious level.

Understanding why we eat as much as we do and why we eat what we eat is important. If we understand what drives us to eat as we do, we can eat less, eat healthier, and learn how to communicate with our body well through the food we eat.

Making decisions takes mental energy. Think of how much more likely you are to succumb to temptation at the end of the day

---

[27] Wansink, Brian. *Mindless Eating: Why We Eat More than We Think.* New York: Bantam Books, 2006. Print.

[28] "Mindless Eating: The 200 Daily Food Decisions We Overlook - Brian ...." http://journals.sagepub.com/doi/abs/10.1177/0013916506295573. Accessed 16 Aug. 2018.

compared to the morning. Our brain, being efficient, likes to find ways to make fewer decisions or to make decisions easier. So, to make decisions easier, our brain relies on external cues for making decisions on the food.

For example, an interesting study was done on chicken wings. Students at a party were allowed to take their pick from a variety of different chicken wings. The students were given a bucket to place their chicken wing bones in when they finished eating. Half the students had their pile of chicken wing bones removed from their table periodically throughout the evening. The other half did not.[29]

The group that had the bones removed ate significantly more than the group that continued to see their pile of bones throughout the night. Folks who could not see how much they had eaten ate more. They didn't have the same external cues impacting and informing their brain and cueing them to stop eating.

Out stomach is bad at determining when we are full. It simply takes too long to send feedback up to our brain and let us know that we've eaten enough.

We rely on things like our plate size, the people around us, and other environmental cues to let us know when we should stop eating.[30]

We overeat not because of hunger but because of the people, packaging, and cues that surround us. Step numero uno is to realize that our choices on food are impacted by the world around us. Step two is to figure out which environmental drivers are impacting you. Then, the tough part (which we will cover soon) is to go about changing things.

Mindlessness vs. Mindfulness

Have you ever eaten the last stale, store-bought cookie? Even if you don't really like cookies and find the store-bought ones too sweet?

Why do we overeat on food that doesn't taste amazing?

---

[29] "Collin R. Payne's research works | New Mexico State University, New ...." https://www.researchgate.net/scientific-contributions/13339592_Collin_R_Payne. Accessed 16 Aug. 2018.
[30] "Plate Size and Color Suggestibility: The Delboeuf Illusion's Bias ... - Jstor." 11 Nov. 2011, https://www.jstor.org/stable/10.1086/662615. Accessed 16 Aug. 2018.

As we eat, we look for our environment to tell us when to stop.

This is mindless eating. When we eat without stopping to think about why we are eating the food in front of us, we become a victim of our environment.

How much you eat will be driven by things like the amount folks around you are eating, the size of your plate, or the packaging and labeling of your food.

One of my biggest passions is to awaken inside people a deeper understanding of how they communicate with their bodies. I want people to understand why they do the things they do and how much of an impact they can have on their health.

I see so many folks floating through life allowing work, daily responsibilities, and the cares of the world to dictate exactly how they live their life.

But we can't be victims of circumstance. We need to be changers instead of blamers.

I'm tired of seeing folks get to retirement and not be able to enjoy it. I'm sick of seeing people wind up in the hospital with preventable diseases, being told it's just a part of old age. I'm done with people not understanding how to communicate well with their body through the food they eat.

So wake up!

Awaken to the drivers behind **why** you live like you do. Only then can you truly change things.

Be mindful. Pay attention to the world around you.

It's a beautiful world. We just need to sharpen our senses to see it clearly.

Start With Slowness

The process of mindfulness begins with slowing down.

It's impossible to be mindful of the food we are eating when we eat it rapidly. But when we slow down, taking time to think about each bite, each meal, and the experience we are having, mindfulness becomes natural.

Start today. Slow down. Pause between bites. Chew your food and enjoy the experience.

Here are two things for you to try:

1.   Be the last person at the table to finish.

2.   Set a time for a meal. Paul, slow-eating ninja extraordinaire, sets one for 20 minutes.

Chronic Speed Eaters

Hi, my name is Matt.

I am a chronic speed eater.

I grew up with plenty of food on the table at my house, most of it being really healthy. But for some reason, I've always eaten really fast. I am often the first one done with my meals. I don't always give my stomach enough time to catch up with how much I've eaten.

I think my speed eating was one of the big reasons why I was overweight growing up.

As I got into high school and college, I became more serious about wrestling. I was exercising two to three hours every day, doing some of the most intense wrestling-style workouts. For this reason, I was able to maintain a relatively lean physique even while overeating and eating quickly. But once I stopped wrestling, I didn't stop eating too much and eating quickly. Within 6 months of my wrestling career being over, I gained about 20 pounds. I topped the scale at nearly 200 pounds, which was the heaviest I've ever been.

I knew I needed to do something about my weight. The worst part was that I was a personal trainer at the time and supposed to be a model of health. But really the only thing I was modeling was the fact that I could get away with eating way more than I should, not eating healthy, and exercising in abundance to burn off calories.

I decided I needed a coach.

I started a year-long online program where I became the client. The program emphasized eating slowly and eating to 80% full as anchor and keystone habits.

As I started eating to 80% full and eating slowly, I gradually started losing weight. I stopped having indigestion every night after dinner. I started to enjoy the process of eating more and question why I'd been eating so fast in the first place.

I don't understand why we eat so fast. Maybe it's because we're stressed, and taking in a bunch of food all at once relieves stress.

Starting to eat to 80% full and eat slowly was the second major turning point in my healthy living journey. The first was starting to diet at the age of 11, and the third and most recent was starting to care about the quality of food I eat and how it communicates with my body.

Although these two habits were the toughest for me to master, they made the biggest impact on my life.

Simple But Not Easy

Eating slowly is simple: Chew your food longer. Take a breath between bites. Lose weight and keep it off. Easy, right? Not in our society. Drive-throughs, eating while we look at our phones, and eating at our desk while we work is the norm.

It is time to bring your focus to how quickly you're eating. It is a very important step in understanding the cues of our body.

We are often rushed when sitting down to eat. We scarf down our food out of busyness or distraction. Either way, we wind up burpy and hungry soon after.

There are many health benefits to gain from slowing down your eating:

- Digest things better... Use those chompers!
- Eat less
- Quality time with great people
- Ease with weight loss and maintaining a healthy weight
- Enjoy food more

Why Do I Need To Eat Slowly?

First, and most importantly, eating slowly will help you eat less food. Better said: Eating slowly will help you eat the right amount of food. The hormones in our stomach that sense fullness and send the signal up to our brain for us to stop eating take time to get going. If we rush through meals and barely chew our food, we will end up eating more food than we need.

Eating slowly sets us up to create a better environment for health.

Second, eating slowly helps to digest our food properly. An important component of digestion happens in the mouth. Our teeth grind food and salivary amylase breaks down carbohydrates. If our food doesn't spend enough time in our mouth, it's more likely to cause problems in our gut.

If we're able to digest our food fully, we will be less likely to have gastroesophageal reflux disorder (GERD) or problems with our weight.

Eating slowly also helps us to enjoy the food we eat. The slower we eat, the more time we have to savor the richness, flavor profile, and pure enjoyment that food can bring. Food was created to be enjoyed.

Although this habit is simple, it's very difficult. If you embark on the journey of eating slower, you'll be met with social gatherings where you're distracted, eating on the go as you rush to work, or trying to feed your toddler or grandchild while you eat.

It's challenging, so don't beat yourself up when you mess up. Your goal is simply to eat a little slower!

Tips For Slowing Down

Knowing you eat too fast is easy. Speed eating is something that most of us have been doing our entire adult lives. It's rooted deeply in our habitual centers of the brain. This is likely why fast-food restaurants are so popular.

I traveled to Kenya in the summer of 2016 for a physical therapy rotation and mission trip. I was amazed by how often the Kenyans stop to eat and rest. They are really quite inefficient from an American point of view! We would have a big breakfast each morning, head into work around 9:00 (ish) and take a break for tea at 10:30. A break after an hour and a half of work!

What I loved about their culture was that they were present and in the moment during meal times. They knew there was more to life than work. Taking time in the day to sit and break bread with family and friends was a must.

Airplane Mode

When you eat, put your phone on airplane mode.

It's easy to numb our brains by scrolling through social, reading an article, or watching cat videos while we eat. This makes savoring our foods and being mindful challenging.

This has been a tough one for me. I like to be as "efficient" as possible. I put "efficient" in quotes because multitasking while I eat doesn't help me to get more done in the long run.

It's tempting to whip out my phone and scroll through the endless loops of Instagram, email, "Saturday Night Live" videos, watch a little *Stranger Things* or something else while I eat.

I see incessant phone use as a bad habit. Now my phone goes into airplane mode anytime I sit down to eat. This gives my eyes a break and allows me to recharge before I tackle what's next in my day.

Minimize Distractions

Distracted eating makes overeating much more likely. When you eat with the TV on, your phone in front of you, or other distractions, it makes it more likely you'll eat more food.

Turn off the TV, set your cell phone in another room, and don't eat while driving, when possible. Setting up a simple, distraction-free environment will allow you to focus on what you're doing now: enjoying your food and monitoring how your body feels.

While growing up, my family was huge on eating dinner together. The TV was never allowed to be on, and as cellphones became a thing, we had to leave them away from the table. I thought it was annoying growing up, but now it's a rule in the Klingler house, too.

Be present, be in the moment, and take time to savor the food you eat and the people you eat it with.

Put Your Utensil Down Between Each Bite

This was and is surprisingly hard for me. Taking the time to put your utensil down after each bite is a great way to take more time between bites. If you look around, you'll notice many folks shoveling food into their mouths as quickly as they possibly can. (Guilty!)

Instead, take the time to breathe between each bite and make sure you have fully swallowed the previous bites before taking your next one. I've heard we should aim to liquify our food, and I think this is a great rule of thumb.

Set A Minimum Number Of Chews Per Bite

Start simple: 10 chews for each bite you put in your mouth. Like all new endeavors, this may feel nearly impossible, but once you practice, you'll get better quickly. To become a slow eating master, you need to get up over 20 chews per bite (CPBs).

Saliva plays an integral role in digestion of our food. The more time food spends in your mouth, the longer you get to experience the sensations of tasting the food and the better you'll be able to digest it. Win-win!

Use Different Utensils

Using a smaller or different utensil is like outsourcing your slow eating. This will help you eat slower without you thinking about anything. Try using a smaller fork or spoon (baby spoons abound at my house) or even chopsticks!

Depth Of Digestion

Tiny food particles make for one happy stomach.

As we've come to see, the food we eat is a language that communicates with our body. If our food is not broken down adequately, the body will receive less nutritional communication. Eating slowly is part of improving nutritional communication inside our body and cells.

Dr. Richard Mattes, a professor from Purdue University, explains, "Particle size [affects the] bio accessibility of the energy of the food that is being consumed. The more you chew, the less is lost and more is retained in the body."[31]

Spit Shine

The moment we start chewing, and even when we think of or see pictures of food, the process of salivation begins. Saliva lubricates

---

[31] "Chew more to retain more energy -- ScienceDaily." 15 Jul. 2013, https://www.sciencedaily.com/releases/2013/07/130715134643.htm. Accessed 26 Sep. 2018.

our food so it can slide down our throat. Better yet, it contains important enzymes for digestion. One such enzyme is salivary amylase, which is important for digesting carbs. If you miss this step in digestion or don't linger long enough, digestive upset is likely to occur and issues will arise.

Less Gas And Bloat

My wife and friends can attest to the benefits of my slow eating. Before I started eating slowly, I was burpy and gassy much more often. I didn't get the nickname HazMatt for nothing!

The human body has about 100 trillion microorganisms in the intestines. This is a number 10 times greater than the cells in the entire human body. Crazy, right?

The reaction between these bacteria and undigested foodstuffs can lead to gas, bloating, diarrhea, constipation, abdominal pain, cramping, and other digestive problems if your food is not chewed up enough.

Slow down. Your gut bacteria and friends/family will thank you.

Next we are going to take a small turn and talk a little bit about a place that you can easily fall off the slow-eating train:

The Buffet Mindset

Buffet eaters consume an average of 42% more calories than those at regular restaurants.

The reason? We want to get our money's worth!

I think this is the same psychological phenomenon that is at play when folks eat food in the work staff room simply because it's free.

I know if I pay for all-you-can-eat sushi, I'm going to get my money's worth. "$25 for sushi lunch? These people are going to lose money on me!" is the mindset of many.

The same thinking can be applied to holiday gatherings. (I always seem to overeat at these. Curse you, cocktail weenies!)

Sympathetic Speed Eating

Rushed eating makes it much more likely you'll tap into the sympathetic (fight-or-flight) nervous system. This is part of the reason why digestion is so difficult when we eat quickly. Speed eating makes it difficult to be in tune with subtle hunger cues in our body because we're in survival mode.

When in the sympathetic mode, your body doesn't care about your digestion, immunity, or your feelings. This makes it impossible to know when to stop eating. It keeps your body working — and eating — on "autopilot."

This leads to us missing out on the pleasure and joy that can be derived from eating good food. When we eat slowly, we taste subtle things, we feel slight differences in texture, and we fully experience the food in front of us. Food is a gift meant to be enjoyed. There's no way we can enjoy the food we eat when we're shoveling bite after bite in while scrolling through Facebook or answering emails.

So slow down. Stay in the moment and be present. Dim the lights if you want. Light some candles and turn on some music. Give your brain a chance to catch up with the fullness signals in your body. Give your brain a chance to get in tune with what's happening as you eat.

Plan

Eating slowly can be a struggle for many people. We are used to being in a rush all the time, and eating can sometimes feel more like a chore that we have to fit in — and generally one that gets done while we are working on something else! I'm so guilty of this! I almost always eat breakfast and lunch while working, reading, or doing something else. Dinner is often the only meal where I am just with my family. But even then, I'm trying to wrangle a toddler into eating things he doesn't really want while he incessantly asks for more "brea!" ("bread" in Cooper talk).

If eating slowly is important to you, you'll take time to plan for slow meals. How we spend our time is a great indicator of our priorities. Making any habit an integral part of your life requires a shift in priorities.

Maybe you know you have a lunch meeting conference call on Tuesday or that you have to run straight from the office to soccer practice on Thursday night. In either instance, you may want to block off some time for eating. Simply giving yourself a 30-minute window where you have nothing to do except eat a meal could be life-changing for you.

Take a look at your calendar right now. Plan out when you're going to eat all of your meals tomorrow. Really: Stop reading and look at your calendar.

Are you done?

How long did you block off?

Were you realistic with how much time you'll have for eating?

If you find yourself saying, "There's no way I can spend 20 minutes just eating in the middle of my work day," you're exactly the type of person who needs to slow down and take a break.

I think we fool ourselves into thinking we need to work all the time. In reality it's probably about 20% of our working hours that generate 80% of the results. What I mean by this is that I think you'll be more efficient and feel better and actually get more important things done if you take a break to eat your meals. I'm totally preaching to myself here. Just yesterday, as I was writing a few pages before this, I was contemplating watching an episode of *Stranger Things* season two while eating my lunch. But I started feeling very convicted by my own writings, so I decided to just eat. I couldn't believe how many times I found myself thinking about grabbing my phone, iPad, or doing something. I've been conditioned to always be doing something. Do you find yourself doing the same?

Can I Just Eat Whatever I Want?

You know the answer to that if you've been reading this book in order. Even though eating slowly will help you eat less, if you are putting less garbage in your system, it doesn't make things much better.

We still want to communicate well with our body through the quality of food we eat.

But this does give you the ability to eat a burger from The Back Abbey (one of the best burgers in LA), enjoying it slowly. You'll find yourself getting full before you finish the burger. At that point, you stop.

Intuitive Eating

Eating intuitively simply means listening to your body as you eat.

When you eat intuitively, you don't need to count calories, weigh your food, or pay a caloric exercise penance.

I've seen way too many clients and well-meaning dieters try to lose weight by simply eating less of the crappy foods they are already eating.

Instead, we need to change our mindset towards food. We need to think deeply about the food that we're eating, instead of just eating it because we want to lose weight.

We need to eat food that communicates well with our body. We want to create an environment for our internal milieu to thrive. We already have everything we need programmed into us to be healthy and fit.

Intuitively, it helps us to get in touch with how our body is responding to the food we're taking in.

Think Before You Eat

Next time you reach for the ice cream in the freezer, ask yourself why.

Trust me, this will be hard. Everything inside your reactive brain will be screaming to shut down the high-level thinking required to understand why you're reaching for the ice cream. This is called metacognition. Metacognition is getting outside of our own brain and looking in. It's thinking about how we're thinking.

Ask yourself, "Am I actually hungry, or looking for emotional reasons, or eating out of habit?"

I find that I'll tend to eat something sweet for dinner more often on nights when I've had something sweet the night before. This is because it has become a habit. A routine. My brain thinks after dinner it's time for something sweet. That's my motive and my driving factor behind why I'm reaching for a piece of dark chocolate or some ice cream after dinner.

I think we intuitively know which foods treat our bodies well. The only way we can hear what our body is speaking to us is to eat slowly, mindfully, and to pay attention.

The Mental Game Of Eating

Physical and mental health are tightly linked.

If we can get our "heads in the game," we will think about the process of weight loss much differently.

Think about creating a good nutritional environment of communication for your body, and weight loss will happen.

Focus on behaviors, like eating slowly, instead of just outcomes, like weight loss, and you'll be much more likely to succeed.

Emotional Eating

How often we eat and what foods we eat are often driven by emotions. If we are frustrated or upset, we will often go for high-sugar, processed foods. These foods offer a quick rush of dopamine to our brain, releasing feel-good chemicals and "fixing" what our brain determines is the problem.

Fatigue

When we are tired, our willpower will be lower. High-sugar foods are an attempt to get quick energy.

The solution is to get seven to eight hours of sleep each night in a cold, dark room. (More on this in the sleep chapter.) If sleeping through the night isn't possible, take an afternoon nap to recharge your batteries.

Lonesome

Food can be a source of pseudo-comfort when we are feeling alone. If you live alone, are in a bad relationship, or are going through a recent life-change, it's easy to grab some ice cream and sit in front of the fridge while you eat.

Surround yourself with people. Get out to the gym, a coffee shop, or even the library.

Hangry

During my time writing *Salubrious*, my wife was either pregnant or breastfeeding. Let me tell you from first-hand experience, you don't want to let a pregnant or breastfeeding woman go more than a few hours without food!

We tend to become emotional, irrational, and to eat more when we do eat if we are overly hungry.

I think a great solution is to have a healthy-fat snack before you get to the point of hangry. Try some salted, roasted nuts before going out to dinner if you tend to overeat.

Frustration

This is the same thing as being stressed or lonely. We are seeking security and comfort and sometimes try to find it from food. Sadly, food is a poor source of comfort because it is short lasting and tends to make people feel guilty after they have eaten a particularly unhealthy meal.

Solution: If you're having an angry moment (like Miles Finch in *Elf*), find other ways to cool down and stay away from unhealthy foods. Get out for a long walk, exercise, write down how you're feeling, or confront the situation head-on if you can.

Willpower

We have all heard the diet advice of "eat less and move more." While this is a great, simple tip, there is a lot more to losing fat. One big aspect is willpower.

Willpower is defined as "the ability to control oneself and determine one's actions." I'm sure the concept of willpower is not new to you at all, but the application when it comes to fat loss might be.

Willpower is a finite resource. We need to work it like a muscle to keep it strong and engaged. It also depletes as we use it throughout the day.

The first way it can be depleted is through self-control. The stronger the urge to do something, the more willpower will be burned during the struggle. Especially when we are on a "diet," these choices can add up quickly throughout the day.

Willpower is depleted throughout a day by making decisions. These can range from simple things, like what clothes you want to wear in the morning, to important, complicated decisions made at work.

As you can see, these may not have anything to do with your food or "diet" choices. The more decisions you make in a day, the less willpower you will have left over to make good food and lifestyle choices later in your day.

You've likely had one of those mentally draining days and gone home only to choose a quick, unhealthy meal. This shows that relying on willpower alone is not a sustainable approach to long-term fat loss.

Now that we know that just relying on willpower will not be the easiest way to reach our goals, we must learn how to conserve willpower for those times when we need it.

Willpower Is A Limited Resource

Unfortunately, temptation is inevitable. Sadly, the more we strive to eliminate temptation from our lives, the more desirable those temptations become. For example: Eliminate sugar and dairy from your diet, and you'll dwell on a the wonders of vanilla bean ice cream all day. You become more aware of the various food temptations during the day if you go on a diet.

You'll notice the apple tart your wife decided to buy at the local bakers all the more when you're following a carb-conscious healthy-fat plan. (Thanks, Nicole.) :)

Willpower is the ability to say no to the apple tart when your mind says you need it.

The more we dwell on eating the apple tart, the more likely we are to cave.

An interesting study was performed on willpower. Two groups were given five minutes to think out loud. One group was told to suppress thoughts about chocolate and another was not given direction.

Then researchers offered both groups chocolate. Like a six-year-old who is told no, the chocolate suppressors ate twice as much.

It's the same with dieting; the more we resist a certain food or food group, the more appetizing it becomes.

So how can we shift this mindset and get the results we want?

Eliminate Choices

You've probably heard how Mark Zuckerberg wears the same thing every day. He does this in an effort to eliminate choices. He understands that we only have a finite amount of choosing ability.

The more we tap into our ability to choose, the less likely we are to make good choices.

An intriguing study was done on Israeli judges. The study wanted to see what factors impacted the judges' decisions in a hearing. It was hypothesized that things like race, severity of the crime, and personal biases would be influential.

Shockingly, none of the above mattered. The main factor that influenced the judge's decision was the time of day. Yup, that's right: A criminal is more likely to have a favorable outcome based on the time of the hearing.

The judges gave drastically more favorable hearings early in the morning and following each of their food breaks. The more decisions the judges had to make, the less likely they were to think rationally.

You're the same. The more choices you have to make during the day, the more likely you are to eat half the bag of kettle-cooked BBQ chips when you come home from work.

You've got to eliminate choices. Always have a plan for what you will eat during the week and day. If you know your mid-afternoon snack is going to be two cups of popcorn, you won't have to think twice about heading to the vending machine for a bag of chips.

If you already have dinner planned out and the ingredients are purchased, you'll be much less likely to grab In-N-Out on your way home.

If you have a workout plan scripted exercise-by-exercise, you won't just do a few sets of biceps curls and head home.

I would also recommend not wasting your energy making unnecessary choices throughout the day. Don't price-shop for the cheapest shampoo. Pick out your clothes the night before.

Add, Don't Subtract

The way we set up Village is additive. We give tons of new recipes and workouts to try. Yes, you aren't supposed to veer off the plan, but we haven't demonized any specific food groups.

When you diabolize a food group (gluten, for example), it creates the mind-occupying thought process we discussed above.

Focus instead on *adding* to your diet. Add in protein or vegetables with every meal. Find new and unique ways to cook the foods you are adding in.

First Things First

Your willpower is strongest early in the day. This is why doing your most important task for the day early in the morning is essential.

If you're looking to get stronger, you should be hitting the gym in the morning before work.

Want to lose weight? Make planning out your food for the day in detail the first task you conquer each morning.

Looking to get new inspiration or motivation? Make reading a self-help book or watching inspirational videos the first thing you do each morning.

Bottom Line

Willpower is limited. Start early. Start small. Add instead of subtracting. Find ways to eliminate choices. Go crush it!

The Almond Challenge

Next, I have an exercise to help you practice eating slowly.

Eat an almond... really, really slowly.

At some point in the next few days, grab a handful of almonds. (If you hate almonds, any nut will suffice.)

Book 15 minutes with no interruptions or distractions to complete the following task. If you can't find 15 minutes, you should evaluate your busyness and schedule.

1. Set your almonds out in front of you and look at them.

Inspect one of them. Notice how it is unique and different from the others.

2. Smell it.

Does it smell almondy? Salty?

3. Put it into your mouth.

Let it sit there. Notice the texture with your tongue. Take your time.

4. Bite it.

Notice what happens as you chew. Does the taste change?

Swallow and repeat.

Observe carefully.

What kind of things did you notice? What things did you taste? Did you find this really difficult? If you found it challenging, it's a good indicator that you likely rush from meal to meal without being mindful of the food you're eating. If you truly take the time to do this exercise, it can be a powerful difference maker in your thinking about the food you eat.

Diane

Diane is the ideal client. She takes everything we say at Village to heart — and then some. When we asked our clients to start eating slowly and more mindfully, she jumped on board.

As a speed eater, eating slowly was tough for her at first. But as time went on, she got used to it. She became a slow-eating ninja working her way through meals at the pace of a turtle. In the process, she started losing weight, being more mindful of her food, and even finding joy in eating.

Diane has started to communicate well with her body. She moves often and moves well. She eats good food in the right amounts, slowly and to 80% full. She would be the first to admit she's not perfect. But she's certainly not going back to her old ways!

CHAPTER 8: FOOD JOURNALING
AND WEEKLY PLANNING

Question: What did you eat for dinner three days ago?

Write it down.

Of course, if you can't remember, don't worry.

Most people can't remember. And when they do remember, they get it way wrong, even though they'd swear they're right.

Research that compares people's recall of their food to what they actually ate shows that people can underestimate their intake by up to 1000 calories a day.[32]

That's just human nature. We're horrendous at remembering.

That's why we don't rely on memory. We write stuff down.

Awareness Brings Change

Knowing more about your food intake and your eating decisions makes you more self-aware. More self-awareness means you're in charge of your environment.

You can celebrate smart choices. Tackle any potential challenges. And make any necessary adjustments as you walk the path to a better body and better health.

Record what you eat each day. This habit is pretty simple.

---

[32] "Why Calories Count: The Problem With Dietary-Intake Studies - The ...." 28 Mar. 2012, https://www.theatlantic.com/health/archive/2012/03/why-calories-count-the-problem-with-dietary-intake-studies/254886/. Accessed 26 Sep. 2018.

Use some method of recording every food and drink item you put in your mouth.

You can use pen and paper.

You can snap a shot with your cell phone. (Try using something like Evernote or DietSnaps, which allows you to annotate a photo.)

Or use an online tracker like Myfitnesspal.com. I think this is the easiest.

Monday – 8:13 AM
- 2 eggs
- A few handfuls of spinach
- Half a bell pepper
- ½ onion
- 1 Tablespoon Ghee
- ½ apple
- 1 cup of coffee

Or it could be something like this:

Monday – 11:42 AM
- About 1 fist of full-fat yogurt, ½ cup strawberries

Food Recording Tips

The goal is awareness.

I really don't want to create a calorie obsession. You are simply writing down everything you eat in an attempt to understand how you are communicating with your body.

You can weigh and measure food as you get the hang of this. Or you can simply keep using our hand-based portion sizing (e.g. one fist of veggies, etc.).

Record what you eat immediately.

Memory is very untrustworthy. Don't try to reconstruct your food intake in the evening or the next day; you'll likely forget a few things or misjudge the portion sizes.

Here's where a notebook or your smartphone comes in handy. If you're at work or out to lunch, just pull out a small pad of paper and quickly jot down your food. Or snap a photo. (Pretend to be a gourmet foodie and say it's for Instagram.)

Record everything. Don't omit things just because you are ashamed of having eaten them.

In other words, if you consume it, it must go in the food journal.

If you eat a Reese's peanut butter cup at 4:13 p.m., it's OK. Really. Just write it down.

From time to time, we all eat things that don't help us achieve our goals. And that's fine. Keep it real and don't lie to yourself. You simply want to know what kind of environment you are creating for yourself.

What To Look For In A Food Journal?

So now you have this amazing food journal. It's time to start looking at the environment you're putting into your body.

Are you implementing the above habits most of the time?

If not, set out to create change in your nutrition environment in the way you think will be most helpful.

The Weekly Plan

One of the key habits of the most healthy Village clients is some form of weekly planning.

In our house, Nicole writes down the planned breakfast, lunch, and dinner each week. Then she creates her grocery list based on her plan.

This certainly is subject to change. We may end up having dinner with friends, having extra people over and not having leftovers for lunch, or deciding to eat out. The important thing is not that you follow the plan 100% of the time. The important thing is that you took the time to write things out. You'll be so much more successful over time if you do this exercise repeatedly.

Plan for success and adjust to changes along the way.

Sandra

Sandra has been food journaling for the last 18 months while she's been a Village client. She has lost over 40 pounds and has learned how to keep it off. She thought she was eating healthy. It turns out she had some room to improve in her nutritional communication, but more importantly, she was eating too much.

With food journaling, she was able to bring awareness to her portions and see major success!

PART 2: MOVE OFTEN

Dr. Matt Klingler | Dr. Erik Gullen

Physical Retirement

You've likely been saving for retirement for years or even decades.

Each month you have a certain percentage of income allocated to go towards a Roth IRA, 401K, or savings account. You've sectioned off part of your check… You kissed it goodbye and said, "I'll see you in 30 years."

But are you doing that with your health?

How have you been saving for your *physical* retirement?

Are you putting in each day for your physical health you hope to cash in on later in life?

You can invest daily in your physical retirement by creating an environment of health for your body to thrive in.

Simply by reading this book (and making it this far!), you've made a deposit in the "physical retirement" bank.

By making a healthy meal or going for a hike tomorrow, you are making a deposit in the physical retirement bank.

By setting up healthy routines and patterns in your life, you create an environment conducive to a bountiful physical retirement.

One Car, One Body

My first car in high school was a 1989 GMC Sierra. The paint was flaking off, revealing the county water division logo and the GMC's previous life. The car had over 200,000 miles on it and quite a few quirks. Even though the car was an oldie, I treated her well because she was all I had.

When I heard the "one car" analogy below from our client Sarah (thanks, Sarah!), I thought back on my GMC Sierra. Even though I took great care of that car, I would have taken even greater care of it had I known it was the only car I would ever have.

So here goes the analogy:

Imagine if you could only have one car for your entire life. Just one car. What would change about the way you take care of that car? What kind of fuel would you put in it? How much more would you pay attention to the necessary service checks, oil changes, and tire rotations it needed? How concerned would you be when it started showing signs of wear? Cars today are (or at least should be) built to last for decades. Your body is like the one and only car you get for your entire life. You need to steward and care for it well if you want it to last and work well for decades.

Here's the good news: Our joints, muscles, and connective tissues were created to last 120-ish years and maybe more. But because of the way we communicate through the food we eat, the lack of moving often and moving well, inflammation takes hold and things wear out much faster than they should. We have everything we need written into our genetic code to live a healthy, pain-free, and vibrant life. We simply need to figure out how to communicate with our bodies in such a way that we create an environment where our genetic code can be expressed well.

It's so easy to forget the pressing importance of caring for your body and communicating well with it on a daily, weekly, monthly, and yearly basis.

"Motivation doesn't last. But neither does bathing. That's why we need it daily." - Zig Ziglar

This is where this book and community come in. Village exists to constantly remind you, to motivate you, to encourage and push you to invest in your health, to care for your body, and to make it a priority. In our busy world, it's so easy to put your health and body on the back-burner for years or even decades while you handle seemingly more pressing matters like work and a busy schedule with kids activities. I agree that work and family are of the utmost importance. But I would also push back and say you'll be able to better care for those you love, and even be better at your work, when you carve out time to care for your body and your health.

Move Often

Exercise is much more than simply a means to burn calories.

"Exercise is important because it generates signals to build muscle, bone, or other lean tissues instead of unwanted fat." - Catherine Shanahan, Deep Nutrition

I detest shirts that read along the lines of "I Exercise So I Can Eat Pizza!"

To have a healthy view of our body, we need to think of exercise as a means of communicating with our genetic code and something to be enjoyed. We need to see exercise and movement as play. Exercise puts our body in an environment to thrive and live well.

The right type of exercise can even create an environment in our bodies where fat cells are more apt to turn back into muscle or some other more useful tissue.[33]

Exercise builds blood vessels, decreases our sensitivity to insulin, and even reduces the stress hormone cortisol.[34]

Make It A Habit

I had an epiphany today while discharging a physical therapy patient to exercise on his own at home.

I told him to do his exercises four times a week and to have set times at which he did them. Then I told him that if his pain was flaring up to show up at the gym anyway: "Even if the pain is so bad that all you do is sit in the sauna and read the paper... The reason," I continued, "is that the most powerful component of your continued healing is the formation of a healthier habit. Even when you are not exercising a particular muscle, you can still be exercising a habit."

I think this is really applicable for you. Who cares if you are tired, a little under the weather, or experiencing some aches and pains. Maybe you are not going to be able to give 100% to your workout on a given day, but you can and absolutely must give 100% to the habit behind it.

Believe it or not, Village Fitness and the book *Salubrious* are not primarily here to help you exercise three hours a week. We are here to transform your remaining 165 hours into a powerful, habit-

---

[33] "The cellular plasticity of human adipocytes. - NCBI." https://www.ncbi.nlm.nih.gov/pubmed/15900154. Accessed 28 Aug. 2018.
[34] "Deep Nutrition – drcate.com." http://drcate.com/deep-nutrition-why-your-genes-need-traditional-food/. Accessed 28 Aug. 2018.

centered lifestyle, and to do that, we ask for your commitment to show up, rain or shine, for your workouts.

As something of a perfectionist, it can be hard to show up for a workout if I don't feel like it's going to be great because I'm tired or have a stomach ache or whatever it may be. However, showing up for the sake of building a habit gives me freedom to have purpose for the time even if the workout isn't the best.

In other words, the workout is the battle, but the habit is the war. Sometimes you have to lose a battle or two to win a war.

CHAPTER 1: THE LIFESTYLE ATHLETE

YOU Are A Lifestyle Athlete

We're going to start off the Move Often section of the book by talking about the mindset of a salubrious person.

If you want to truly be salubrious, you need to view yourself as a Lifestyle Athlete.

Now, before you start thinking you can't be an athlete because of an injury you have, or not having time to do a competition, stop.

Being a Lifestyle Athlete is more of a mindset than anything else.

The reason we do Small Group Training here at Village is because we wanted to create a team-like atmosphere for our clients. A team has coaches, trainers, experts, and therapists who know what they are doing. A team is there to celebrate difficult parts of life with you. A team is there to go through the valleys and the peaks with you. A team is there when you are frustrated about not losing weight from the last month or when you are dealing with the nagging knee injury that seems to come back too often. A team is there when you hit a new Deadlift PR or when you go to the doctor's office and finally get off statins. A team is there to celebrate and support.

A team could be the people you work out with in Small Group Training. A team could be a group of friends you get together and walk with. A team could be the four other people who run Spartan races with you.

Life is so much better when you can share in the struggle and the joy and victory with a team of people.

In a world where isolation and pseudo-connection via technology are the norm, being a Lifestyle Athlete and being part of a team are very countercultural.

Different Seasons

As a Lifestyle Athlete, you'll go through different seasons.

Athletes train differently when they're in season compared to when they're out of season. When they're training for a competition or big game, they tend to pick up their intensity and train harder. When they finish the game, they may take a few weeks off to let their body recover.

Athletes get injured. They need to take time to heal from injuries, to learn why they got injured in the first place, and to come back even stronger.

Far too many clients we've worked with and people in general do the same exercise routine every week of the year. There's no undulation or variety to what they do.

Variety Is The Spice Of Life

Throughout the course of a year, your training should vary. There should be times when you're training intensely, working towards getting as strong and as fit as possible. Maybe you work towards an event or competition or simply getting stronger on a specific exercise.

At Village, we max test a few times every year. We test our clients' strength on a few key exercises like squats, deadlifts, and bench press. Then we spend a month or two of intense, focused training on those exercises. Then we test again. After this we cycle back to less intense workouts.

There should be times in the year where you are intently focused on changing your nutrition. Through the year, we have various nutrition emphases and focuses for our clients. There are times of the year where we do nutrition challenges, offering an extra amount of focus on certain aspects of nutrition.

There will probably be times when you're battling an injury. It's a normal part of the athletes' lifecycle to get minor injuries because they are pushing the limits. During these times you need to shift your focus from getting stronger and fitter to healing, doing physical therapy, or getting a therapeutic massage.

There will probably be times of the year when you're extra busy and need to set minimums for yourself so that you can still stay fit and progress towards your goals. This would be something like tax season for an accountant, back-to-school time for a teacher, or Christmas for a pastor.

The important thing is to make these seasons short and intense so you can continue to pursue this Lifestyle Athlete journey well.

Purpose

Picture an Olympic skier.

For four-plus years, a big part of their life revolves around preparing for an event. They have their eyes on the prize of making the Olympic team, getting on the podium, or winning a gold medal.

For the Lifestyle Athlete, this looks a bit different.

Maybe it's something tangible like completing a 5k race or beating your hiking time up Monroe Truck Trail here in Glendora. Or maybe it's something like being able to put a heavy carry-on in the overhead bin on your next trip, being able to lift your grandchild without back pain, or having the confidence to take a walking travel trip 10 years from now.

Maybe your prize is getting on the scale and seeing you've lost 20 pounds, or fitting into a certain dress for an event or a cruise.

Maybe your prize is simply finishing the day today and knowing you did everything in your power to set yourself up for success.

When you have your eyes on the prize, you take off the blinders of self-doubt, past failures, and disappointments. You can't have that stuff in your vision, clouding your focus if you're keeping your eyes on the prize.

This is something that should motivate and change your behavior all the time.

Imagine the Olympic skier again. Everything they eat, how they move, their sleep, and their life-routine will be impacted by keeping their eyes on the prize.

For you, knowing you have a prize you're working towards will change the food you eat, the movement you do, and your daily routine.

The Olympic skier wins gold! Do you think they are satisfied and ready to call it quits? Probably not. They are likely looking ahead to the next prize.

So you also, once you get your "prize," will continue to press on. You'll move towards the next goal and then the next. Is this a meaningless journey with no destination? By no means! The fun is in the journey. In this journey you'll not only learn how to communicate well with your body but also how to live a life rich with health and good memories.

Always Wear This Hat

Being a Lifestyle Athlete is not a hat you can take off. It's an identity thing.

Much like a parent is always a parent, a Lifestyle Athlete is always a Lifestyle Athlete. It's part of who you are — 100% of the time.

Deep down, people are carrying the weight of past disappointments and failures.

We need to get deeper, to get through all those layers, to pull things back in order to get through to the heart of a champion.

If you hear cynicism or doubt when you hear this, we are speaking to you.

You are a Lifestyle Athlete.

You were created to be disciplined, enduring, strong, to thrive, to win, to achieve. It's central to who you are.

CHAPTER 2: GREASING THE GROOVE

Maxing Out

A few times a year, we do max testing with our clients.

We want them to see just how strong they are and then see them go through the process of improving over one or two months. Then we test again.

We want our clients to get excited about making changes in their strength on specific exercises. We don't see this as simply a reason for people to get stronger for strength's sake. But rather, max testing is our deliberate attempt to empower our clients to accomplish more in life. We want our clients to be better spouses, grandparents, friends, or co-workers.

We see what we do at Village as much more than simply hosting fitness sessions, helping people lose weight, or helping folks get out of pain. We see what we do as something that helps to change people's lives and the lives of those around them for the better. We see it as our mission to change your environment so you can change the environments of others.

Then We Grease The Groove

To become better at swimming, you need to practice swimming. To improve your tennis backhand, you need to work on your backhand.

To get stronger, you need to practice strength.

Greasing The Groove, popularized by Pavel Tsatsouline,[35] is a technique we use twice a year at Village to help clients get stronger and improve performance in specific exercises.

We want our clients to be excited about their fitness. We want them to come into the gym pumped up to improve on their bench press, deadlift, squat. We want them to feel like they are progressing towards meaningful goals at Village.

Then, when clients hit these goals in community, they will feel a sense of accomplishment. They will feel like an overcomer. This will carry over into life. Like a client said recently, "I now know I am the type of person who does squats, deadlifts, and bench press. Like, that's me." It's pretty cool to see when caring well for one's body becomes a part of someone's life.

Our hope for Greasing The Groove is to make people into not just stronger bench pressers, deadlifters, and squatters, but better parents, spouses, friends, and coworkers.

We want our clients' goals to go deeper than the superficial goals of weight loss or getting stronger. We want our clients' goals to delve into the depths of who they are. We want the workouts our clients do at Village to have carryover into their life.

Let's say at the beginning of the month a client is unable to deadlift their body weight. Then, after a month or two of consistent practice, they can now lift more than their body weight. This is so much more meaningful than just lifting more weight.

When we consistently work at strength and view it as a skill and a craft to master, we will get better, be stronger, and see the carryover into life.

Neurological Strength

Think of water running down a hill. Eventually, water finds the most efficient path down the hill. A rut forms in the hill and you have a stream. Before long, you've got yourself a full-fledged river!

The process of getting stronger works similar to this. As we do the same exercises repeatedly, the same neurons in our brain contract the same muscles, in the same coordinated sequence and pattern.

---

[35] "StrongFirst: The School of Strength." https://www.strongfirst.com/. Accessed 16 Aug. 2018.

Over time, this process becomes efficient and fast. This is called myelination.

Myelination is the process by which a fatty substance forms around the axons of our nerves that allows them to communicate more quickly.

As we age, if left to our own devices, our neurons de-mylenate. One of the best ways to prevent this is through strength training.[36]

How To Get Strong

There are two ways to get strong, and we use both of them at Village. The first is to lift heavy weights and to continue lifting heavier. This causes small tears in our muscles, inflammation, and forces our body to adapt and change as we go through the strengthening process.

The other way is by Greasing The Groove. With Greasing The Groove, we lift lighter weights, more often, and with higher reps to teach our muscles to become more efficient and better at specific exercises. Essentially we are, like Pavel says, "practicing the skill of strength" (imagine a thick Russian accent).

Nicole's Greasing The Groove Journey

My wife, Nicole, practiced Greasing The Groove with pull-ups a few years ago. When she started, she could do a few pull-ups before hitting failure.

Each day she worked out, which was three to four days a week, she would do a few sets of pull-ups well below her maximum level (two to three reps). After a few months, when she tested pull-ups again, she was able to do 10 with ease and fluidity!

One of the keys with Greasing The Groove is **not working to failure**. If you are training to failure three days a week on the same exercises, you are setting yourself up for failure, burnout, and potential injury.

THE WEIGHT YOU USE SHOULD BE MODERATELY CHALLENGING.

---

[36] "The effects of normal aging on myelin and nerve fibers: A review ...." https://link.springer.com/article/10.1023/A:1025731309829. Accessed 16 Aug. 2018.

Start lighter than you think you'll need to go, and then you can work your way up from there as you get used to the GTG type of training.

CHAPTER 3: THE HEART
(STRENGTH TRAINING)

When I was an undergraduate, I had an eccentric professor who taught the core of our exercise physiology classes. His name was Dr. Shaffrath.

I really took a liking to him after our first class, when he stood up on the desk and shouted exuberantly pretending to be a cholesterol molecule or something like that. I don't remember the specifics of the analogy, but I do remember laughing like never before in a lecture.

He also happened to work out at a gym where I was a personal trainer.

One day I walked into the gym and was greeted by Dr. Shaffrath. "Klingler!" he announced. "Come to the bathroom and see this!"

At first I was a little taken aback, but I obliged.

When we got to the bathroom, he proceeded to point at a naked gentleman in his 70s. We were well within earshot of the gentleman, which made it all the more awkward.

"You see, Klingler," Dr. Shaffrath said, pointing at the naked man's backside. "This is what happens when you lift weights. Those are the glutes of a man who has squatted with weight for decades."

The man gave us an odd look and proceeded to put on his clothes promptly. But Dr. Shaffrath kept going. He told me about the horrors of senile sarcopenia and how strength training helps prevent it, all while standing in a locker room full of naked men.

Lifting weights helps us to be able to do the things we want to do and makes the golden years actually enjoyable.

This interaction has stuck with me for years. Now that I've worked in the big hospital system, I've seen how many people are unhealthy, don't exercise, and become victims of the pills, injections, and surgeries the medical world offers as a "solution."

Why You Should Lift Weights

Strong people are hard to kill.

I'm a firm believer that we don't have control over the day that we will cease to exist on this planet. But I think we can have a huge effect on the quality of the years we have. I love the phrase "strong people are hard to kill" because strength training and being strong makes us impervious to many of the common diseases and problems that tend to wreck lives.

When you lift weights, and get strong, you not only improve your circulation, the strength of your heart, and the functioning of your brain, but you also set yourself up to do the things that are important to you for years to come.

You might be thinking, "But my goal is to lose weight. Won't lifting weights make me bulky?"

No.

Strength training is actually one of the keys to you getting the lean, fit, and healthy body you're striving for.

Lifting weights helps to elevate our metabolism long after our workouts are complete.

Because your body will be hard at work to repair the muscle you've broken down during your strength training sessions, it uses up calories as fuel.

Then, as you age, because you're strength training, you maintain your lean muscle mass so you can keep hiking, playing with your grandkids, and walking when you're traveling Europe, or doing mission work in Haiti. Whatever it is that you want to do with your physical retirement, strength training is imperative to make it a reality.

Weekly strength training sessions should be like an automatic deposit into your 401(k) account.

You may not even see the effects of these "deposits" today, but they are an investment in your health long-term. Strength training is going to set you up to be able to have a great physical retirement.

The beauty is, once you start and get into a routine, it's easy to keep going, and some people even find it enjoyable. (Gasp!)

I think one of the keys is to have something you're working towards like the Lifestyle Athlete we mentioned earlier. You need some sort of number or goal to keep you motivated.

It could be something as simple as trying to improve the amount of time that you can do a farmer's carry with 30-pound dumbbells. It could be the weight on your bench press for five reps. It could be getting closer to a bodyweight pull-up. Whatever it is for you, have something to work towards.

Structuring A Workout

Our muscles were designed to work in a coordinated action. Therefore, the exercises we do should use multiple large muscle groups. This is why, at Village, we rarely do things like biceps curls, lateral leg raises, or triceps extensions. It's not that these are "bad" exercises per se; it's just that we understand that people are busy and don't have endless time to work out.

We need to do the exercises that will give us the most bang for our buck.

I'm guessing you don't want to spend hours in the gym each day, right?

To get stronger, or maintain strength as you're trying to lose weight, it's important that you have enough recovery time between your workouts. We recommend about 48 hours between training sessions. But if you're someone who only has between the days of Monday and Thursday to get three workouts in, it's fine if you do Monday, Tuesday, and one on Thursday. This way, you get three days to recover over the weekend and you come back for the next Monday ready to rock.

It's also important to note that there really aren't any "good" exercises. Our body doesn't understand what squats, pull-ups, or lunges are. What any body understands is the amount of tension placed upon the muscles, how long the tension is on the muscles, and where the joints are in relation to each other.

91

Our body doesn't understand how much weight we use either. Using 70 pounds on bench press with poor form and a fast tempo is likely not as effective as using 50 pounds, a slow tempo, perfect form, and feeling it in all the right places.

So, as a client does a lunge, I'm always asking them whether or not they feel their glutes firing, if it's challenging, and if it's causing pain. If the exercise is challenging to the correct muscles, with enough to get sufficiently tired, I consider it a "good" exercise. Simply doing squats or lunges and not having a purpose for them is pointless. This is why I think it's so important to go to the gym with a plan and pursue your workout passionately instead of scrolling to Facebook and Instagram between sets while you try to figure out what to do next.

Your workout should be a time dedicated and focused on investing in your health. You should have a set amount of time that you allow yourself for strength training each workout session. For example, set a timer on your phone for 30 minutes and have a goal to get through as many sets as possible with amazing form on six different exercises you chose. This will keep energy high during your workout and keep you motivated.

Some of the best workouts I've ever had have been when I was crunched for time and knew I needed to be disciplined in order to get my workout done. Some of my most lackadaisical workouts have been when I knew I didn't need to be anywhere after the workout so I could take my time.

What About Machines?

I don't recommend using the machines at the gym. The problem is that they force you through a confined movement path. This isn't natural for your body.

In fact, the back extension machine has been proven to be one of the highest compressors of spinal disks when extending backwards. Dr. Stuart McGill has done research linking lower back health more to endurance and less strength or flexibility.[37]

---

[37] "Spine flexion exercise: Myths, Truths and Issues affecting health and ...." http://www.backfitpro.com/spine-flexion-exercise-myths-truths-issues-affecting-health-performance/. Accessed 26 Sep. 2018.

How Many Reps Should I Do?

First, it's important to note that our body doesn't understand reps. What it understands is the amount of time you place it under tension when you're exercising. Therefore, 5 reps done with a slow, 4-second lowering and a 2-second lift, will take just as much time as 12 reps done relatively quickly. These two will have a similar amount of tension placed on your muscles. But just for your enjoyment, I will lay out the recommended rep ranges below.

1-5 Reps: Power, strength, fat loss
5-12: Strength, fat loss, muscle building
13-20: Endurance, strength

What I don't like about defining certain rep ranges to categories like endurance, strength, fat loss, or power is that any range of strength training will yield some measure of each of those categories. If you do 20 reps, you'll increase your power, burn fat, and get stronger. Would using 5 reps of a heavier weight be better for fat loss than 20 reps of a lighter weight? I think so. But doing *something* is so much better than spending your time trying to get it perfect.

Moving Well With Strength Training

We'll talk more about this in the Moving Well section of the book, but there are a couple important things I want to touch on here. First, it's imperative that you have a good rib-cage position and activation of your tummy muscles when you strength train.

For the ribs, you want to think about bringing your rib cage down before performing any strength training exercise. With exercises like pull-ups and shoulder press, I often see people flare their ribs out as the exercise gets more challenging. This is problematic because you lose most of your core stability and control if your ribs flair. This puts added stress on all of our muscles because they don't have a good foundation to work off of. Think of a house being built on a sand foundation as opposed to a concrete one.

Flared Rib Cage Shoulder Press   **Ribs Down Shoulder Press**

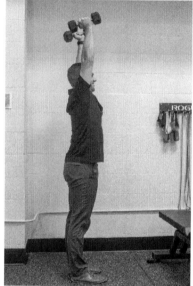

Incorrect   *Correct*

To assess the activation of your core muscles, poke your finger into the area about six inches to the right or left of your belly button. This is your lateral abdominal wall just comprised of muscles by our internal and external obliques and our transversus abdominis. These muscles act like a support belt around our midsection and give us a solid breathing foundation. When we perform exercises like squats, deadlifts, or shoulder press and we use these muscles, our cores get stronger, and muscles like our biceps and quads have a strong foundation to work off. Only performing these exercises without our lateral abdominal wall being activated creates instability and problems with the exercises.

The Basic Six Movements

OK! Now we are on to the big six movements of strength training.

At Village, we structure our clients' workouts based on movements from each of these six categories. Humans are fairly complex and able to move in an infinitely different number of directions and patterns. But, to simplify our lives and to ensure we are hitting most muscle groups in every workout, we recommend breaking things up into these six categories.

Squat

Squats use the big muscles in our legs like the glutes, quads, and hamstrings. When done with good spinal position, they tap into our core stability. Squatting is the most basic and fundamental of human movements. Many babies love to hang out in the squat position. As we age, we squat less frequently.

Squats have practical implications in many areas of our lives. For example, the ability to get up and down off the toilet, and getting down on the ground with your grandkids to play Legos are impacted by our ability to squat. Squats can also assist in our ability to empty our bladder fully, preventing hemorrhoid development, and strengthening our pelvic floor.

Balance: Squat To Bench

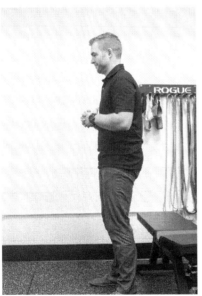
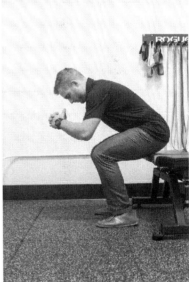

Start   *End*

Fitness: Kettlebell Goblet Squat

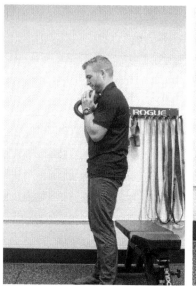 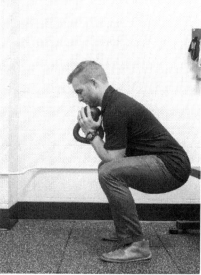

Start   *End*

Village: Barbell Back Squat

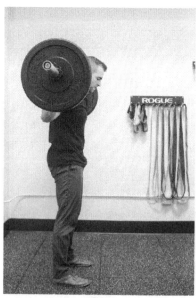 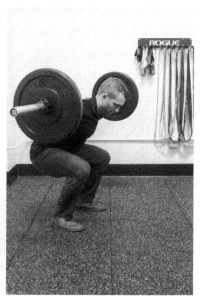

Start   *End*

Hinge

The hinge movements are the most difficult to teach and perform correctly. These include movements like deadlifts and kettlebell swings. The hinge movements are hip dominant. This means that the hips move more than the knees and back.

These exercises usually target the glutes, hamstrings, calves, and back extensors.

When done correctly, they are an integral part of a good training program. When done incorrectly, they can lead to low back pain and other injuries.

Balance: Wall Hinge

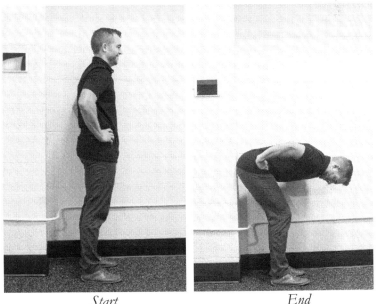

Start   *End*

Fitness: Dumbbell Single Leg Romanian Deadlift

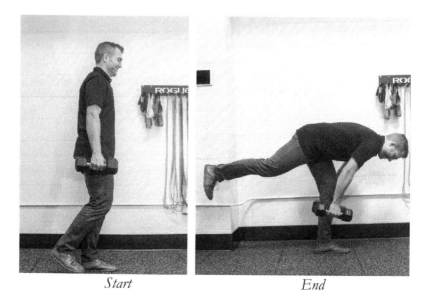

Start   *End*

Village: Barbell Deadlift

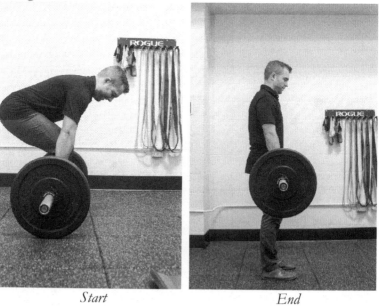

Start   *End*

Lunge

Think of stepping over rocks while on hikes, climbing stairs, and getting up and down from the ground. Lunges develop strong, shapely legs and accelerate our ability to burn fat because of the big muscles used.

We put all step-up and lunging exercises in this category.

Balance: (TRX Reverse Lunge)

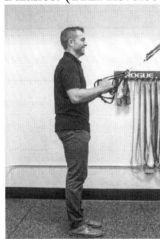 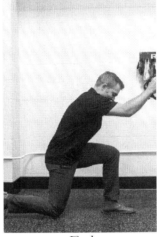

Start   *End*

Fitness: (Bodyweight Reverse Lunge)

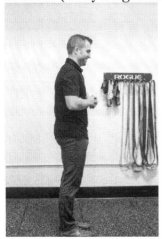 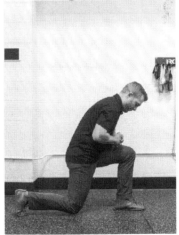

Start   *End*

Village: (Dumbbell Reverse Lunge)

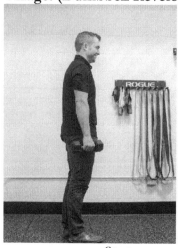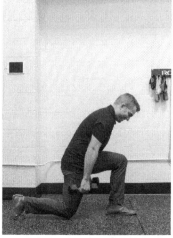

Start   *End*

Upper-Body Push

This category includes anything where the weight is moving away from your body. Think push-ups and shoulder press.

Upper-body push movements usually use muscles like our chest and triceps. At Village, we like to use large, multi-joint muscle exercises like a dumbbell bench press, the shoulder press, or TRX chest press.

Balance: (TRX Chest Press)

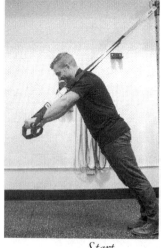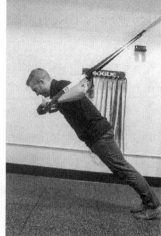

Start   *End*

Fitness: (Elevated Pushup)

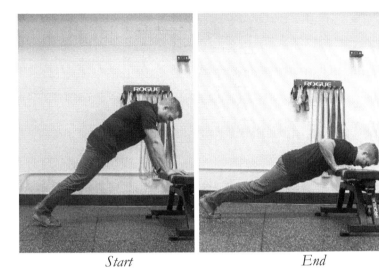

Start   *End*

Village: (Pushup)

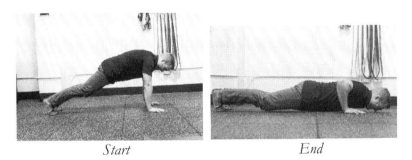

Start   *End*

Upper-Body Pull

When you think of an upper-body pull, think of exercises like pull-ups, single-arm rows, and face pulls. These exercises strengthen the muscles of our back and biceps.

Balance: (TRX Row)

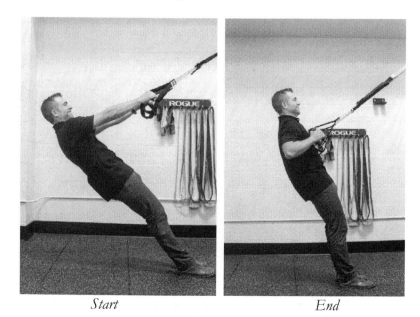

Start   *End*

Fitness: (Band Assisted Pull-up)

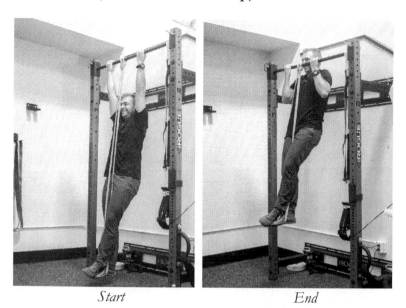

Start   *End*

Village: (Bodyweight Pull-up)

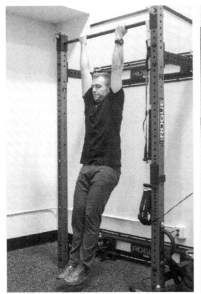
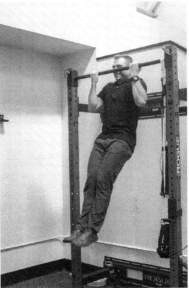

Start   *End*

Twist/Core

The core is central to everything we do as moving humans. It serves as the link between our upper and lower body. Core strength and coordination have been linked as an integral component of preventing low back pain and living a healthy life.

Balance: Side Plank Bottom Knee Down

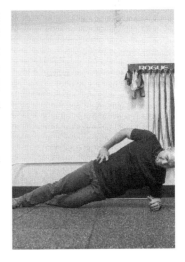

Fitness: Side Plank   **Village: Side Plank**
                                    Top Leg Lifted

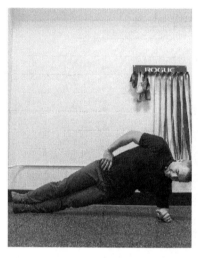 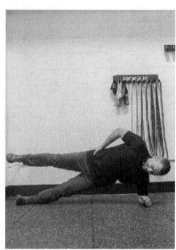

How To Get Started

At Village, we do something called the Village Fitness Experience. It's a four-week journey towards understanding how to communicate well with your body. We help clients lay the foundation for communicating well with their body through movement in our Small Group Training program.

If working out at Village isn't an option, I suggest finding yourself a coach.

Finding A Coach

Finding a coach is a daunting task. The fitness world is a broken place. If you don't know what you're looking for, you'll be an easy target for quick-fix weight-loss schemes and protein-shake diets.

The fitness industry is unregulated. Anyone can call themselves a "personal trainer." Anyone can claim to be a nutrition expert and give nutrition advice. Thankfully there are many qualified people in the fitness industry who know what they are talking about and have coached hundreds of people.

Based on my experience coaching people for over a decade and working in numerous health and fitness settings, the following are what to look for in a good coach. My hope is to help you ask the right questions and find a place that will help you achieve your goals.

Do They Look Like A Coach?

If you work in the health and fitness industry, you should practice what you preach. There are personal trainers who are out of shape, don't exercise, and set a poor example for their clients. Although they may have head knowledge, they lack the personal motivation to back it up.

But just because someone looks ripped doesn't mean they know how to coach. If a specific program works for a personal trainer, it doesn't mean it will work for you.

Side note: One of the most lean and ripped trainers I've ever known ate a strict diet of three Carl's Jr. Spicy Chicken Sandwiches each day. Was this effective for getting him lean? You bet. Was it healthy? Heck no. Think of all those PUFAs!

I don't think a trainer needs to have six-pack abs. I've never had a six pack and yet I consider myself a good coach. But your trainer should look like he or she works out.

Credentialing

My first personal training certification was a course I took at home at the age of 18. Looking back, I can't believe I was certified to coach people on their health and fitness after reading a single book and getting at least a 70% on the test. Yikes!

I think a college degree in some sort of exercise science is a great start. It shows that the coach is serious about their craft.

Ask Good Questions

I am always amazed by how few people want to know my credentials or background as a coach before signing up for our programs at Village.

I encourage you to ask good questions:
- How long have you been a coach for?

- What is your current understanding of what it will take to get to my goals?
- What is your philosophy on habit change?
- What's a realistic time frame to reach my goals if you coach me vs. going at it alone?
- What makes you worth more than the trainer down the street?
- Can you tell me stories of people like me you've helped see results?
- How often will you follow up with me outside of training sessions?
- How will the training program be presented?
- What sort of guarantee will you offer if I don't see results?

Affordability

Here are a few questions that can help you consider whether a trainer is within your budget.

Can you afford to work with the coach long-term? If they charge $100 per session for one-on-one training, can you afford the $1,200 a month to work with them?

At Village, our Small Group Training program provides a one-on-one-like experience at a fraction of the cost. It's pretty cool!

Ask good questions about price. Would the coach be willing to write you a program for the days you are not with them? What are the costs for nutrition coaching?

Talk To Others

Find someone who has worked with the coach you are considering. Ask them good questions about their journey.

A good coach can be a life-changing addition to your health or a draining, money-wasting time suck. I suggest you ponder, consider, and make sure you choose well before diving in head-long.

Melody

Melody started working with our team at Village a few years ago. When she started, she was dealing with chronic back pain and frustrated by how her body looked and felt.

After about six months of consistent strength training, she started noticing positive changes! Her back no longer bothered her. She was seeing more tone and definition in her arms, butt, and legs. Her belly fat had all but left, too!

Her husband commented that she looks better than ever and seemed to have a renewed sense of confidence! "Don't ever stop working out there!" he told her one day.

Now Melody is able to do a full pull-up without assistance. This is an impressive feat of strength.

Because of how our Small Group Training program is structured, she felt the coaches were able to give her the attention she needed to keep her body safe as she got strong and lean. She found immense value in Small Group Training, comparing the quality of coaching she received to buying something from Nordstrom that will last a lifetime.

CHAPTER 4: THE APEX
(INTERVAL TRAINING)

Anaerobic exercise is so difficult and mind consuming that you can think of nothing else while you're doing it. Imagine sprinting up a hill (or away from a mountain lion). This type of exercise should burn.

This high-energy, short-burst type of training creates an amazing communication with your body. Once the exercise is over, your body goes to work to prepare you with what you need to do that type of exercise again. You'll need more lean tissue and less body fat. You'll need to be faster, more springy, and strong.

Thankfully we don't need much of this type of training to thrive (10 to 30 minutes a week). Just 15 minutes of ALL-OUT cycling intervals over a 2-week period produced amazing gains in muscle power.[38]

Our body is like an eager student, sitting in the front row of class, waiting to be told what to do next. When stimulated to become more fit and build muscle, it will go about converting fat cells into more useful tissues to be ready to perform again. It will increase your metabolism to be ready to create more energy.

At Village, the APEX is the high-energy, metabolic conditioning portion of your workout.

---

[38] "Six sessions of sprint interval training increases muscle oxidative - NCBI." https://www.ncbi.nlm.nih.gov/pubmed/15705728. Accessed 27 Sep. 2018.

APEX-style training should not only spike your heart and get you sweating, but should make you feel like you can accomplish other things in life.

Interval training alternates between periods of high-intensity exercise and low-intensity or rest. The spiking of intensity forces your body to generate energy rapidly and then recover. The repeated on and off will improve markers of cardiac function, spike metabolism, and make you fit in a hurry.

Interval training is metabolically expensive. This means it takes lots of energy for your body to make these intervals happen.

In this chapter, we'll spend time considering the benefits of interval training, the different styles of interval training, and then give a few examples of interval workouts. This is by no means an exhaustive resource on interval training, as whole books can be and have been filled by information on interval training.

Fat To Muscle

When we eat too much, especially vegetable oil and sugar, our body needs to find a place to store the extra energy. So it finds stem cells in the body and converts them into fat cells. The excess food energy creates the signal and communication for your body to store excess calories in the form of fat.

The opposite is true of un-doing this. If you create the right communication and signals, your body will seek to turn fat cells into more useful tissue like muscle, nerve, and bone.[39][40][41]

Research shows that 10 to 30 minutes of intense exercise per week (APEX-style interval workouts) can provide the necessary cellular information for the conversion of fat cells into tissue like muscle, bone, nerve, blood vessel, and tendon.[42]

---

[39] "Transdifferentiation potential of human mesenchymal stem ... - NCBI." https://www.ncbi.nlm.nih.gov/pubmed/15084518. Accessed 26 Sep. 2018.
[40] "Reversible transdifferentiation of secretory epithelial cells into ...." https://www.ncbi.nlm.nih.gov/pubmed/15556998. Accessed 26 Sep. 2018.
[41] "The cellular plasticity of human adipocytes. - NCBI." https://www.ncbi.nlm.nih.gov/pubmed/15900154. Accessed 26 Sep. 2018.
[42] "Insulin-resistant subjects have normal angiogenic response to aerobic ...." https://www.ncbi.nlm.nih.gov/pubmed/26038468. Accessed 26 Sep. 2018.

Efficiency

For the busy person, interval training is a time-effective way to get an effective workout. Most folks think that they need to spend hours in the gym in order to get an effective workout. But with interval training, just 10 minutes can get your blood pumping and create the communication you need to achieve the results you want.

Interval Formats

Negative rest

In a negative rest format, you work for longer than you rest. For example, a 30-second interval on the bike followed by 15 seconds of rest. These types of intervals are great for getting a higher volume of time at the high level of intensity.

Example:
Rowing Machine
5 minute warm-up
1 minute all-out row
30 seconds easy or rest
Repeat 10x
5 Minute cool-down

Positive rest

In a positive rest interval, you rest for longer than you work. These types of workouts are great for when you're looking to train your body's ability to recover and work at a maximum intensity.

Example Workout:
Battle Ropes: 45 seconds all-out
1 minute rest
Squat To Press: 45 seconds all-out
1 minute rest
Step-ups: 45 seconds all-out
1 minute rest
Rowing machine: 45 seconds all-out

Variable Work: Rest

Example 1:
Work for as long as it takes to complete 20 ball slams.
Rest for 30 seconds.
Battle ropes for as long as it took to complete the ball slams.

Example 2:
Rowing machine until you get your heart rate to 170, keep it there for 15 seconds.
Rest until your heart rate comes back down to 120.
Repeat until thoroughly cooked.

Tabata
"Ciabatta?" clients respond when I ask if they have heard of tabata.
Tabata intervals or 20-seconds-on, 10-seconds-off were created by an exercise physiologist with the last name "Tabata."

Example: Hardest 4 Minutes Of Your Life
20 seconds: Barbell Front Squat
10 seconds: Rack bar, take a few breaths, get set for next set
Repeat 8x
This one is downright nasty. I've done this with 115 pounds on the bar and turned my legs into utter jello in 4 minutes.

Get Unconventional

Don't be confined to using a bike, elliptical, or running as the only means for doing interval training. Dumbbells, barbells, kettlebells, or just about any implement can be used for interval training.

Dumbbell Complexes

A "complex" involves moving in rapid succession from one exercise to the next using the same set of dumbbells throughout. These are a great way to get a cardio or interval-style workout without having to use a machine.

Bicep Curls   2,4,6,8,10,12

Front Squat	2,4,6,8,10,12
Burpees	2,4,6,8,10,12
RDL	2,4,6,8,10,12
Mt. Climbers	2,4,6,8,10,12 each leg

Sled Push

If you have access to a sled, it's one of the most brutal and effective lower-body training tools out there. Simply pushing a sled across the grass, gym floor, or outside is an amazing challenge.

Hill Sprints

Simply find a hill and sprint up it. Walk down. Repeat.

How Often?

Don't overthink it. Keep it intense. Keep it short. I like to tell people they need to get to the point where things are burning and stay there for a few minutes, multiple times each week. A minimum of 10 minutes and a max of 30.

Too many exercisers do either no interval training or too much.

Workout places like Orangetheory, Soul Cycle, or boot camps tend to be entirely interval-style workouts. Although these workouts are fun, you're communicating such high intensity with your body, it will lead to breakdown. Add in a poor diet and you have a recipe for injury disaster.

Strike a healthy balance. Keep interval workouts short and intense and reap the benefits of a healthier, leaner body.

CHAPTER 5: THE WIND DOWN (STRETCHING, YOGA, FOAM ROLLING)

At the end of a Village session, we Wind Down. This includes stretching, breathing, foam rolling, and a point of finality for the session.

When it comes to stretching and foam rolling, there is so much conflicting information. Things like you need to stretch before and after every workout or you need to be foam rolling each and every night.

After getting my doctorate in physical therapy, working with thousands of patients, and training in the fitness industry for the last 10 years, I've developed my own opinion.

A good warm-up should be similar to the workout, get you physically warm, and fire up your sympathetic nervous system. A good cool-down should bring you back into a parasympathetic state.

Notice I didn't say anything specifically about stretching, foam rolling, or yoga. That's because these are tools to be used in specific cases for specific cool-downs.

A Wind Down should be gentle. I see far too many people doing the reach-forward hamstring stretch. It may feel good, but what you are stretching is really the ligamentous and muscular integrity of your lower back (not a good thing). Plus, most folks need stronger and more active hamstrings (even if they feel tight).

At Village, we always work on breathing during the Wind Down. We all need to breathe better. (More on this in the Breathing section.)

"But My Hips Feel Tight"

Just because a muscle feels "tight" doesn't mean you should stretch the heck out of it.

Take the hip flexors for example. You may have heard that everyone has tight hips because we sit too much.

This is true. But stretching your hip flexors can create its own set of problems, like laxity of your ligaments.

Integrity

Our bodies were created with a muscular tension built in. This tension serves to keep our joints in the right position as we move through life.

When you constantly stretch your hamstrings by reaching forward towards the ground, you're not just stretching the hamstrings but also the muscles, ligaments, and tendons of your lower back.

Foam Rolling

I'm fine with people foam rolling.

Foam rolling should be viewed as a self-massage tool. That's really all it is.

Massage is great for relieving muscular tension and activating the parasympathetic nervous system.

If you spend a few minutes foam rolling before bed, it can be a great nightly routine to tap into the parasympathetic nervous system.

Do I Have To Stretch After I Work Out?

Nope.

I think you'll be just fine if you skip on stretching after a workout.

All of the talk about muscles feeling less sore, more mobile, or less likely to become injured when you stretch after a workout is based on little to no scientific evidence.

You should, however, do something that helps restore a parasympathetic state before leaving a workout. This could be as simple as walking around for a few minutes or working on breathing with your feet on the wall.

How To Actually Get More Flexible

I'll let you in on the secret to how gymnasts get so flexible. But I'll warn you first that many gymnasts suffer from chronic injury and pain years down the road because of their super-flexibility.

You have to stretch for a really long time under a low load.

Think about your hip flexors. If you sit for 8 hours a day with your hip muscle in a shortened position, the 30 seconds of stretching your hip flexors 3 times a week after your lifting workouts probably isn't going to change anything.

If you really want to get more flexible, and I suggest you take time to think about WHY you're trying to make something more flexible, you need to go about it the right way. Gentle and slow. The rule I use is 5 minutes 5 times a day.

A Favorite Village Wind Down

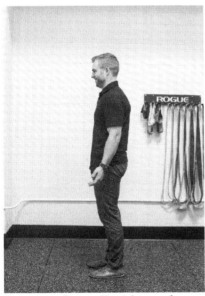

Start standing tall with good posture.

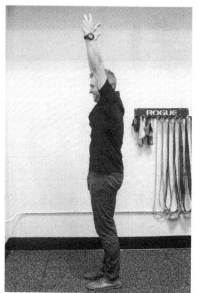

Inhale through your nose, lifting your hands overhead while keeping your ribs down.

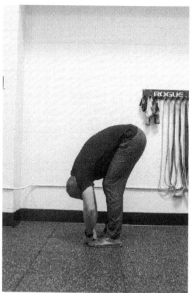

Exhale through your mouth, bringing your arms down near the floor.

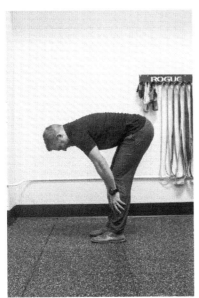

Inhale, sliding your hands up your shins.

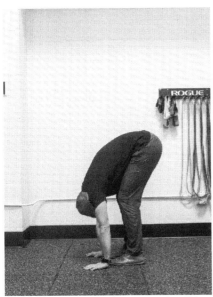

Exhale, reaching down again. Place your hands on your mat.

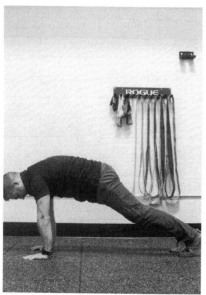

Step back into a pushup position.

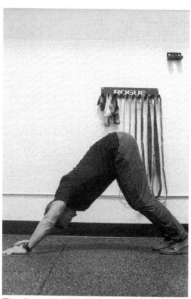

Push your hips up and back into a down dog stretch. Take a few breaths here in through your nose and out through your mouth.

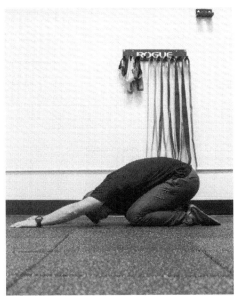

When you're ready, drop your knees down to the mat and rock your hips back into a child's pose stretch.

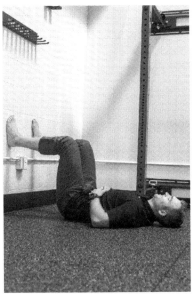

Finish the Wind Down with supine breathing.

CHAPTER 6: CARDIO

The single most important thing to know about cardio is that you don't HAVE to do it.

There. I said it.

I've released you from the bondage and slavery that most people feel to the treadmill.

There is a common misconception that we need to and have to do cardio to achieve our goals of losing weight and being healthy. I hear so often from folks struggling to lose weight that if they could just run more, the weight would fall off. This is almost never the case.

There are a bevy of ultra-marathon runners with beer bellies who can attest to the fact that a plethora of cardio does not guarantee a lean physique.

What Do You Consider Cardio?

There is ample crossover between the aforementioned interval training and strength training with cardio.

But for our purposes, we will define cardio as a single activity like biking, running, walking, or hiking done for a prolonged period of time (greater than 10 minutes).

Exercise For Calorie Burn Is Silly

If you exercise to burn calories so that you can eat more, you are fooling yourself.

You can burn about 500 calories with an hour of riding a bike. Then, you can put it all back in with 30 seconds of cookie eating.

Cardio, strength training, and interval training are important not because of the amount of calories you burn but rather because of how they communicate with your body. These things create an environment for your cells to thrive.

When you exercise, it signals to your heart, lungs, and brain that they are needing to be healthy and vibrant in order to do the work again.

How To Get What You Want Without The Treadmill

But just about any goal you want to achieve can be realised in the absence of cardio.

Want to be leaner? This can be done through strength training and diet.

Want to have better health markers? Again, diet and strength training can get you there.

This brings us to the question of **"Should you do cardio?"**

Here I think the answer is yes.

I think you should find something you enjoy and make it an integral part of a healthy routine.

You Need To Feel It

Your exercise needs to be tough enough to get you breathless, to make your legs and lungs burn, and to push you to your limits. The level of exercise should demand that you're present in the moment and mindful of your movement.

Try to feel which muscles you're intending to work. If you're running, get in tune with your calves. If you're cycling, feel the burn in your quads.

Cardio Has To Be More Than Just Losing Weight

A pastor friend of mine runs a few times a week and memorizes scripture while he runs. At first, his running was a tiresome slog, but now it has become a somewhat enjoyable part of his weekly routine.

For me and my family, cycling is a cardio activity that brings us together and has created some of the most fun memories of my life.

Currently, I ride my bike or run a few days each week. My gym is also my work, so I find getting outside and moving my body is one of the most refreshing and enjoyable parts of my week.

Find something meaningful to you. Maybe it's a hiking or walking group. It could be a race you're training for.

The Benefits Of Cardio

"A bigger heart, more blood, less stress, and vessels bud." - Dr. James Shaffrath

Dr. Shaffrath was a professor of mine when I studied Exercise Biology at UC Davis. His short poem about the effects of exercise on the human body has stuck with me.

A Bigger Heart

The size of our heart is a great indicator of health.

The heart is responsible for pumping blood through our body. When we exercise, it signals to the heart that it needs to become stronger and able to pump more blood. So, in the presence of communication like this, the heart becomes larger and more voluminous.

More Blood

More blood won't make you a better vampire, but it will help your heart function better, keep you healthier, and make chronic diseases less likely.

When you do cardiovascular exercise, your body goes about retaining more blood in circulation. With more blood in circulation, your circulatory system becomes more efficient. This means less stress on the body when you're at rest and exercising. With more blood, you can circle oxygen to your tissues with ease!

Less Stress

This isn't the kind of stress relief you feel when the kids go back to school after summer break. Here we are talking about hormonal stress.

When we exercise, stress hormones like epinephrine and cortisol are released in response to exercise.

Exercise is a form of stress. It's a good stress called a eustress. But it's still a stress. As we become more fit, this stress lessens and we become better exercisers.

This also has carryover into other stressful parts of life. Hello, big work project!

In response to stressful situations at work or home, you'll respond by releasing less stress hormones if you've been doing cardiovascular exercise than if you were not training.

In other words, cardio keeps a fellow (or lady) mellow.

Vessels Bud

As we become fitter, we need ways to get more blood to more tissues faster. The bigger heart and increased blood supply mentioned above are a great start. Now the vessels in our muscles and other tissues bud and increase in number to dump extra blood into our tissues.

Again, this means we will be more efficient and healthier.

How Should Cardio Fit Into My Routine?

Most days of the week, you should be moving. This could be a daily walk, a bike commute to work, or simply an active job where you are on your feet.

You should also plan a few longer, more intense cardio workouts like a bike ride, run, or hike.

The real key here is to find something you don't absolutely detest. If you hate running, for goodness' sake, don't run! If you love riding a bike, ride a bike.

For me, riding a bike is one of the most mind-clearing, relaxing, and refreshing parts of my week. My office is at Village. I'm surrounded by a gym for 40-plus hours a week. Strength training, although an important part of my weekly routine, usually makes me start thinking about business and ways to make Village better.

Cycling, on the other hand, is freeing. So I ride my bike. I don't ride to be lean or for the health benefits necessarily. But those are nice bonuses.

Find something you love to do, find good people to do it with, and make it a habit.

CHAPTER 7: RECOVERY AND SLEEP

We decided to put the Recovery and Sleep section in the part of the book on Moving Often because recovery and sleep are an essential component to being able to have the energy to move often.

Sleep creates an environment where our body can repair, rebuild, and make sense of all the good communication you've given it from food and movement.

As I write this, I currently have a six-week-old. Although my wife, Nicole, is awesome and often lets me sleep through the night, we are still woken up multiple times each night by our baby. My thinking is less clear, my workouts less focused, and life a bit fuzzier than before baby.

If you find yourself feeling burned out, tired, and unable to perform in the office, gym, or at home, it may be due to your sleep quality and/or quantity.

If you go to the doc's office and tell them you have a sleep problem, most will simply prescribe a side effect-laden sleeping pill and send you home. Although I'm sure there is a time and place for sleeping pills, I think the medical world doles out sleeping pills much too quickly and instead should focus on improving sleep through other means.

Our bodies are meant to sleep well. If we are not sleeping well, there is likely something off in the way we are communicating with our body.

We live in an overly busy and stressed society. Far too many people are addicted to stimulants to get them going in the morning and through the day. Then at the end of the day, they need to unwind with a glass of wine or a beer (or more than a glass). Instead of allowing our body's natural hormonal regulation of our sleep-wake cycle, we rely on drugs like caffeine and alcohol.

Although we can't control how fast we fall asleep or how long we stay asleep, we can certainly set ourselves up for a good night's sleep by doing a few things well.

If you want to feel better, live longer, lose weight, and thrive, a good night of sleep is one of the most effective tools to get there. I'm going to lay out some of the best research on sleep as well as my own practical experience.

Sleep Is Foundational

No matter how often you move, a lack of sleep will eventually catch up with you. I've seen clients who are working out every day of the week and eating well struggle to lose weight simply because they are only sleeping five hours a night.

What's Sleep?

"Sleep is a naturally recurring state of mind and body, characterized by altered consciousness, relatively inhibited sensory activity, inhibition of nearly all voluntary muscles, and reduced interactions with surroundings."[43]

With our eyes closed and our consciousness altered, sleep restores energy, regenerates tissues, and prepares us to tackle another day.

During sleep, we progress through five phases. The average person takes 90 minutes to complete each phase. When we are awakened often during the night (like with a newborn), it's difficult to get the appropriate amount of time in each phase.

Why Do I Need To Sleep?

During sleep, the body goes about to build, repair, and regenerate. Important functions like immune system health,

---

[43] "Sleep - Wikipedia." https://en.wikipedia.org/wiki/Sleep. Accessed 27 Sep. 2018.

metabolism and hormonal balance, and brain function can only happen during sleep. We can't survive without sleep.

How To Sleep Better

1. Dark, Sleep-Only Room
The bedroom should only be used for sleeping (and sex). Keeping the bedroom specific to sleep, as opposed to Netflix binges and work chats, will help create the brain association that your bedroom is for sleeping.

The room should be dark. Like *really* dark. Even the smallest blue light should be omitted. Nicole and I will cover any blue lights (like on our sound machine) with tin foil taped over the light. Yeah, we are serious about our sleep. Any light, even a very small light, has been shown to decrease our body's drive to sleep.

2. Create A Sleep Ritual
Start your sleep ritual in the morning. Ideally you should wake just prior to the sun rising. This is one of the best ways to improve sleep. By getting up within the same small time frame each day, you set your circadian rhythm up for success.

Then start your day with a routine.

For me it's coffee, prayer, reading, and then I write or tackle my first most important task for the day. I spend the first 45 minutes to hour of the work day deeply immersed in something meaningful. For the past three months, it's been writing this book.

Having a two-year-old and a newborn make this difficult. Some days the routine gets thrown for a loop and simply doesn't happen. That's OK. Simply having the routine in place and returning to it as many days as possible has set me up for long-term success.

3. 10 Hours Before Bed, No Caffeine
"The single most important factor in winning your mornings and owning the day is to get up 15 minutes earlier and work on your number-one priority before anyone else is awake."[44] - Craig Ballantyne

Craig Ballantyne came up with the numbers for the next few sleep points. He calls it his 10-3-2-1-0 formula for winning the day. All the numbers revolve around bedtime, and I think they present a helpful formula for creating your own set of sleep "rules."

The first, "10 hours before bed, no caffeine," is fairly simple. Caffeine is a stimulant. Far too many people use stimulants in excess to stay wired during the work day. Then at night they use depressants, like alcohol, to calm down. This "works," but it's a terrible solution. When you drink, especially more than a single drink, it causes your sleep cycle to be thrown off (more on this in the next point).

Caffeine in moderation (1 to 3 8-oz. cups of coffee per day) is fine depending on your tolerance levels. But have more than this and you'll soon feel the effects of central-nervous-system fatigue and burnout.

If you have a 9 o'clock bedtime like me, you'll need to have your last cup of coffee at 11 a.m. It takes about 10 hours to clear all caffeine from your bloodstream.

This rule may need to change for those who are more sensitive to caffeine. For me, I am super sensitive to caffeine and alcohol (#lightweight). But my wife, Nicole, can have a latte at 5 p.m. and go to sleep at 9, no problem.

4. 3 Hours Before Bed, Stop Alcohol And Food Consumption

Alcohol impairs our sleep-wake cycle and disturbs restful sleep. Our body is really good at taking us through the stages of sleep, but alcohol throws a wrench in the system.

If you drink too closely to sleep or too much, you may fall asleep quicker, but your sleep quality will suffer.

Alcohol before bed impedes restorative sleep and memory processing. This is essentially altering your ability to process all the amazing communication you've given yourself during the day.

Limiting yourself to one drink and making sure it's at least three hours before bed should help to mitigate or prevent these effects.

[44] "The Ultimate Guide To Biohacking The Perfect Night's Sleep." 16 Jul. 2018, https://drjohnrusin.com/the-ultimate-guide-to-biohacking-the-perfect-nights-sleep/. Accessed 27 Sep. 2018.

Food should be limited just before bed as well. When your body doesn't have time to process the food you eat before bed, it can lead to blood sugar crashes in the middle of the night, waking you up.

5. 2 Hours Before Bed, No More Work

This should probably happen long before two hours before bed, but two hours is the bare minimum if you want restful sleep.

It's really important for our brain to have the chance to shut down and do a "reset" before the start of the next day. If you are always working or thinking about work, it will be difficult to get meaningful work done or be present with your family during non-work time.

As a small-business owner, this is tough for me. I want to be available to handle problems at all times so they can be solved quickly. But I've found that this comes at a cost not just to my family life but also my ability to work effectively.

One of the reasons I've been able to write this book well is through taking downtime and not thinking or talking about work for a few hours before bed.

6. 1 Hour Before Bed, No More Screen Time

Melatonin is an important hormone that helps facilitate sleep. Blue light, like that of a cell phone, screen, or TV, has been shown to reduce its secretion.[45]

Researchers at Harvard also suspect that blue light may have a negative impact upon some types of cancer, diabetes, cardiovascular diseases, obesity, and depression.[46]

I recommend getting a bit obsessive about blocking blue light. Tape tin foil over any and all blue light in your home. Get serious blackout curtains. Create yourself a sleep dungeon!

---

[45] "How Technology Impacts Sleep Quality | Sleep.org."
https://sleep.org/articles/ways-technology-affects-sleep/. Accessed 10 Sep. 2018.
[46] "Blue light has a dark side - Harvard Health." 13 Aug. 2018,
https://www.health.harvard.edu/staying-healthy/blue-light-has-a-dark-side.
Accessed 10 Sep. 2018.

You can put your phone on "night-shift" mode or something similar to block blue light, and this may help. I have mine set this way from 7 p.m. to 6 a.m.

7. 0 (Number Of Times You Should Hit The Snooze Button)

Confession: I hit snooze once this morning. But that's much better than what I used to do!

The general principle is to set your alarm to get up when you want to get up — and actually get up then. Spending an hour in the morning hitting the snooze button is not only a waste of precious morning time, but you are also not getting restful sleep.

8. Read Fiction Before Bed

I have yet to find any scientific research on this one, but it works well for me.

All day long my brain is working to solve problems at work, manage a two-year-old, and make decisions. At the end of the day, I just don't want to think anymore.

You can watch TV to zone out, which takes care of not thinking, but the blue light will likely keep you awake.

Or you can read or listen to fiction to give your brain something else to think and focus on rather than dwelling over the events of the day and thinking about the next day's events.

When I was in physical therapy school, I went through a period of time where I struggled to fall asleep. I would lay there thinking about all the things I needed to get done or go over muscle origins and insertions in my head.

So I convinced my wife that we needed to start listening to *Harry Potter* on audiobook. She obliged, and pretty soon we were hooked. Every night we would spend 15 to 20 minutes listening as we fell asleep. Immersing myself in the magical world of *Harry Potter* helped my brain turn from thinking about the worries of the day to becoming enveloped in a story.

You can also read. I recommend reading a real paper book (they still make these). If this isn't feasible, you can read on a Kindle or iPad, but remember to turn it to "night-time mode."

My favorite fiction books are the *Kingkiller Chronicles*, *The Stormlight Archive*, and, of course, *Harry Potter*.

9. Get Vitamin D

The sun is our body's only means of producing Vitamin D. It helps regulate our circadian rhythm and facilitates good sleep.

We need sunlight early in the day. Research shows that people who get sunlight within the first few hours of the day fall asleep easier at night.

We need direct sunlight. One of the best means for the rays of the sun to enter our body is through our eyes. The eyes have blood vessels very close to the surface of our body.

Attempt to get 15 to 20 minutes of direct sunlight per day without sunscreen or sunglasses on. After that, you can lather up and be confident that you got enough sun to keep your melatonin centers happy as a ray of sunshine.

10. Move Often

Here's another reason to move often: better sleep quality.

Research has found that early morning exercise (taking the dog for a walk) can help us fall asleep better come nighttime. Strength training, on the other hand, helps us stay asleep for longer, as our body works to repair and regenerate so it can come back stronger.[47]

11. Supplement With Magnesium Before Bed

Magnesium is a common mineral found in the human body.

Experts say about half of Americans are not getting enough magnesium and are deficient.[48]

"This is a bonafide anti-stress mineral that offers many more benefits, including that it can alleviate premenstrual syndrome (PMS) symptoms, reduce blood pressure, boost performance, relieve inflammation, prevent migraines,

---

[47] "What Time of Day to Exercise for Better Sleep | Sleep.org." https://www.sleep.org/articles/exercise-time-of-day/. Accessed 27 Sep. 2018.
[48] "Magnesium Deficiency Symptoms, Causes, Risk Factors, and More ...." 9 Feb. 2017, https://www.health.com/nutrition/magnesium-deficiency. Accessed 27 Sep. 2018.

improve blood sugar levels, fight against depression, enhance sleep quality and promote relaxation."[49] -John Rusin

Increasing magnesium levels in our body can decrease stress, reduce leg cramps, and help us sleep better.

I recommend the supplement Calm, which you can buy on Amazon or at Sprouts.

Top 10 Magnesium-Rich Foods Based on Magnesium Concentration:[50]

- Spinach, cooked — 1 cup: 157 milligrams
- Swiss chard, cooked — 1 cup: 150 milligrams
- Dark Chocolate — 1 square: 95 milligrams
- Pumpkin seeds, dried — 1/8 cup: 92 milligrams
- Almonds — 1 ounce: 75 milligrams
- Black beans — 1/2 cup: 60 milligrams
- Avocado — 1 medium: 58 milligrams
- Figs, dried — 1/2 cup: 50 milligrams
- Yogurt or kefir — 1 cup: 46.5 milligrams
- Banana — 1 medium: 32 milligrams

(*Note: mg values are according to the USDA)

12. Sleep In A Cold Environment

When we fall asleep, our core temperature lowers. If the environment we are in is too hot, we will struggle to fall asleep.

The optimal temperature for sleep is between 60 and 67 degrees Fahrenheit.[51] That's cold!

You can also use a fan to promote coolness and a light sheet or   blanket.

13. Breathing Exercises

[49] "The Ultimate Guide To Biohacking The Perfect Night's ... - Dr. John Rusin." 16 Jul. 2018, https://drjohnrusin.com/the-ultimate-guide-to-biohacking-the-perfect-nights-sleep/. Accessed 27 Sep. 2018.

[50] "10 Magnesium-Rich Foods That Are Super Healthy - Healthline." 22 Aug. 2018, https://www.healthline.com/nutrition/10-foods-high-in-magnesium. Accessed 27 Sep. 2018.

[51] "Best Temperature for Sleep | Sleep.org." https://www.sleep.org/articles/temperature-for-sleep/. Accessed 27 Sep. 2018.

Balloon Breathing

With a ball between your knees and your feet on the wall, your body bent to the left, inhale through your nose. As you exhale, dig your heels down into the wall and squeeze the ball. Inhale through your nose, holding this position. As you exhale, lift your right foot off the wall. Holding this position, you're going to blow up the balloon with your exhales. Do 5 breaths into the balloon before releasing.

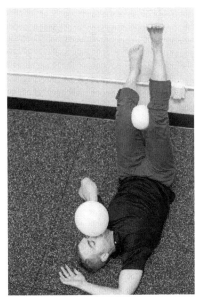

Wall Reach Exercise

With a ball squeezed between your knees and your back on the wall, inhale through your nose. As you exhale, round your upper back, reaching forward. Inhale through your nose without extending up. Perform 5 breaths.

Both of these exercises help correct positional issues and tap into our parasympathetic (rest-and-digest) nervous system.

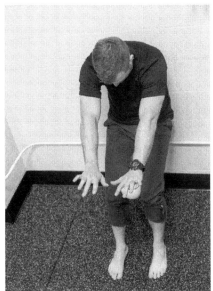

14. Go To Bed Earlier

I get called an old man because I go to bed early. But I am in good company. Arnold Schwarzenegger, Bill Gates, and many other influential minds go to bed early and get up early.

Our bodies were designed to sleep according to the dark times of day. Only in the relatively recent past have artificial lights enabled us to be stimulated to stay up later.

The National Sleep Foundation recommends the following amount of sleep for varying age groups:[52]

- Newborns: 14-17 hours
- Infants: 12-15 hours
- Toddlers: 11-14 hours
- Preschoolers: 10-13 hours
- School-aged children: 9-11 hours
- Teens: 8-10 hours
- Adults: 7-9 hours
- Older adults: 7-8 hours

---

[52] "National Sleep Foundation Recommends New Sleep Times." https://www.sleepfoundation.org/press-release/national-sleep-foundation-recommends-new-sleep-times. Accessed 27 Sep. 2018.

Dr. Matt Klingler | Dr. Erik Gullen

PART 3: MOVE WELL

Dr. Matt Klingler | Dr. Erik Gullen

INTRODUCTION: HOW OUR BODY
WAS MEANT TO MOVE

Our joints were created to last 120 years.

In a world where joint replacements and back surgery are the norm at the age of 50, this is shocking and frustrating.

But the lifestyles we live, the foods we eat, and the way we move (or don't move) cause sub-optimal joint movement, which leads to extra wear and tear on our joints and connective tissue, in addition to pain and arthritis.

If you start to have pain and go into the medical system, you are taking a major risk. Not only is the current solution often to pump people full of painkillers, but patients are also given dangerous labels, which can stick with a person for life.

Consider the 60-year-old woman who has low back pain. She goes to see her primary care physician with her back pain. Her physician has about seven minutes to spend with her. That's certainly not enough time to get to the root of her movement and nutrition issues. So she is prescribed muscle relaxants, painkillers, or anti-inflammatories. None of these address the root problems of the food we eat and the movement we do. But they will often fix the symptoms. Eventually, however, the symptoms will return. At this point an X-ray or MRI may be ordered.

Instead of being told she has normal age-appropriate changes to her spine, she is labeled with degenerative disk disease. Psychologically, this creates a cascade of problems and will lead to this poor woman feeling hopelessly unable to change her problem.

But there is a better way!

Instead of telling people they have degenerative disk diseases and are broken beyond repair, we need to give hope that they can create change through improved movement quality and frequency.

Moving well is equally important to moving often. If we don't move well, we are setting ourselves up for arthritis, pain, degenerative discs, and heading down a road of chronic pain.

The body's compensatory mechanism for abnormal movement is to lay down more bone to stabilize. This pseudo-stability is what leads to degenerative disk diseases, arthritis, and pain.

At Village, we believe you were meant to live well, to move often, and to be free from pain. We want to see grandparents playing with their grandkids, dads enjoying their weekend bike ride or golf game, and retirees able to travel, serve, and enjoy their golden years.

In the coming chapters we will talk about how to breathe well, create good posture, understand pain, and finish with exercises to set you up to move well.

CHAPTER 1: BREATHE

Breathing Is A Top Priority To The Human Body
While this is a fairly obvious concept, its implications are often missed. Before we can explain why, we need to understand a few things about the autonomic nervous system.

The autonomic nervous system works behind the scenes to ensure that all of our vital functions are performed. These functions include pumping blood via the heart and circulatory system, the regulation of resting muscle tone in the musculoskeletal system, digestion, and the acquisition and delivery of oxygen to all of the body's cells in the respiratory system. It's important that it works behind the scenes, because this frees up our conscious attention to more interesting and fulfilling activities (like binging on Netflix).

The autonomic nervous system has two divisions: the parasympathetic, which helps us to "rest and digest," and the sympathetic, which helps us perform "fight-or-flight" responses to danger.

If your body was a castle, parasympathetic means that all the villagers are safe and going about their daily business. The builders are building. The farmers are farming. The artists are painting. The King is tweeting about "Saturday Night Live," and the soldiers are resting up, training, and making sure all the defenses are in place.

Conversely, sympathetic means an army has begun to attack the castle. The builders, farmers, and artists all stop working and lock themselves indoors. The King goes on high alert. The soldiers mobilize to form a counterattack.

Now, to be clear, not every autonomic response is quite this dramatic. The sympathetic response to danger should be proportional to the level of threat. For example, the amount of sympathetic activity provoked by a barking Chihuahua should be considerably smaller than what Jeff Goldblum's character experienced in the famous T-Rex chase scene in *Jurassic Park*.

Both sympathetic and parasympathetic divisions work together in tandem throughout the day.

Consider a typical morning routine. While enjoying your last few minutes of sleep, your body is in full parasympathetic rest and digest mode. Safe.

Your alarm clock goes off, startling your body and provoking a small sympathetic reaction that arouses you from slumber. Danger. You realize that it's still early and decide to hit snooze. Safe.

Your body shifts back to parasympathetic activity as you doze off.

Unfortunately, you miss the next alarm, and when you awake, you look at the clock and realize you could be late for work if you don't hurry. Danger! Sympathetics kick in with a surge of adrenaline to speed through showering and grooming. You have just enough time to scarf down a hard-boiled egg and some berries before getting in your car.

During the commute, you listen to a podcast and forget you're running late, allowing your body to shift back to parasympathetic activity and digesting your breakfast. Safe. These little shifts in autonomic activity help you to get through your day with the right balance of rest and stress.

Overall, humans need to spend most their time in the parasympathetic, rest-and-digest state.

If the castle is always at war, it won't be long before the builders and artists and farmers begin to starve. If there aren't enough soldiers or defenses to overcome the attack, the villagers will have to take up arms and try to help the cause. And won't somebody please think of the children?!

In any case, a castle that is always at war will not become a thriving metropolis. In our bodies, the sympathetic, fight-or-flight state should be reserved for alarming and resolving temporary threats. Most of the time you should feel peaceful and free from danger. However, this is rarely the case.

Chronic stress causes systemic dysfunction in the human body. Without significant time spent nourishing and regenerating cells throughout our bodies, we age prematurely and have symptoms like weakness, fatigue, pain, indigestion, insomnia, frequent illness, irritability in relationships, depression, anxiety... you name it! Unfortunately, getting stuck in a stress state is something of a downward spiral.

First we get stressed. The stress burns us out. We fail to rest and restore. The burnout leads to vulnerability, and more situations become dangerous. We respond to the danger with even more stress and are less able to stop and feel safe enough to rest. Sound like anyone you know? Sound like you? More on this downward spiral later.

Of all bodily functions, accessing oxygen is top dog. Go a few hours without a drink and your tongue will feel dry. Go a few days without food and your tummy will rumble. But go a few minutes without air, and you will literally be on the brink of brain death.

Sound dangerous?

A threat to the respiratory system is Enemy No. 1, and will spur an immediate shift from parasympathetic to sympathetic activity.

Due to our constant physiological dependence on respiration, the body will use the musculoskeletal system, the neurological system, digestive system — any system it needs — to make sure that the respiratory system is working. That's right, if your body is having trouble breathing, it will arrange your posture, your nerves, even the digestion of your Chipotle Chicken Bowl, in a way to facilitate breathing.

Our body's breathing strategy in sympathetic (danger) mode is different from its parasympathetic (safe) mode.

In a safe, resting state, the body uses a muscle called the diaphragm to breathe. This muscle attaches to the front of your spine as well as the bottom, inside part of your rib cage. With the low back and neck muscles relaxed, the rib cage sits in a position that allows the diaphragm muscle to dome. This is its happy place. Breathing in this position looks like gentle inhalation through the nose that causes all the ribs to expand and reciprocate from side to side.

This left-to-right rib cage reciprocation is complemented by our other reciprocating motions, such as walking. It is a beautifully designed, self-regulating system.

By contrast, when the castle is responding to danger, the diaphragm is converted from a villager to a soldier. It is pulled from its respiratory dome shape to become flat and taut to aid in stabilizing the spine as the body gets ready for fight or flight.

Without its primary respiratory muscle, the body must get oxygen somehow! Since the diaphragm can no longer work from below the rib cage to expand the lungs, the neck muscles take over from above, hoisting the rib cage up like a bird cage. Additionally, the muscles of the low back extend the lumbar spine to further lift the rib cage, allowing more lung expansion anteriorly (in front).

If this happens temporarily, there is no problem.

Have you ever been swimming with a friend and had a competition to see who could stay underwater the longest? At first, holding your breath underwater had a surreal, almost peaceful quality to it. But as soon as the oxygen deprivation set in, your body immediately stopped digesting food and directed blood flow and neurological activity to the musculoskeletal system to propel you back to the surface. Once at the surface, you took a few gasping mouth breaths, hoisting your rib cage up, neck muscles bulging out. A few minutes later, oxygen levels had normalized, and you were back to digesting and breathing diaphragmatically through your nose. No problem!

If this happens chronically, there is a big problem.

We live in a world full of stressors, and each of them tells your body to go into danger mode. Whether by environmental pollutants, allergies and asthma, fear of failure, pressure to succeed in career and relationships, accidents, illnesses and injuries — our diaphragms keep getting taken out of a happy, domed shape and getting recruited as a shoulder to defend against danger.

Over time our brains forget what a happy diaphragm even feels like! In a vicious cycle, our low back muscles get tighter and tighter, our upper back and neck muscles get tighter and tighter, and our ribs flare out in front. There is a reason people under stress say things like "I'm suffocating" and why a person finally at peace says they can "breathe a sigh of relief." Stress and breath are intimately connected.

Trying to calm down by "taking a deep breath" is ironic. The respiratory system under chronic stress is suffocating not because of too little air but too much! All those little gasping breaths IN add up, and it becomes increasingly difficult to get air OUT. This is why your ribs stick out in front (above your belly) — the lungs are hyperinflated, like balloons about to pop!

The vicious cycle gets more vicious.

Let's review: Environmental stressors cause the body to shift from parasympathetic to sympathetic activity, and this converts the diaphragm from a respiratory muscle into a postural muscle. When working as a postural muscle for too long, the body faces an additional challenge to breathe. This difficulty breathing due to the lack of support from the diaphragm itself becomes yet another stressor! This additional stress continues to drive the body into a sympathetic state. Eventually, the overuse of low back and neck muscles causes pain and dysfunction in those areas, adding, you guessed it, another stressor.

But wait — there's more!

It's not just low back and neck pain that result from stress-pattern breathing.

The dysfunctional overuse of low back and neck muscles, coupled with hyperinflated lungs and flared ribs, changes the position of the whole body — from your fingertips to your toes. Think of it this way: Your spine, ribs, and pelvis are the house that your shoulders, elbows, hands, hips, knees, ankles, and feet live in. If the house is falling over, it won't be long before the joints that live there fall over, too.

And that's not all! Remember earlier when we talked about the neurological and digestive systems? In a chronic sympathetic state, the neurological system is on high-alert, alarm mode.

Pain receptors become more sensitive than normal, and any injury is not only more painful but also more emotional and memorable. Meanwhile, the digestive system is all but forgotten. Its ability to break down food, absorb nutrients, and move waste out regularly and comfortably all diminish. At first, a person under stress will feel decreased appetite. Eventually, nutrient-starvation will cause appetite to increase without regulation, spurring what is most often referred to as "emotional eating."

Oh, go on! While this section could continue quite a while longer and delve more deeply into all of the dysfunction caused by chronic sympathetic breathing, suffice it to say that it is a root cause of a myriad of health concerns that are often treated with costly surgeries, pills, infomercial supplements, etc. At this point, things may look a little bleak for us, but don't worry.

Let's get into the solution:

Respiration is the one vital function under both voluntary and involuntary control. This is a big deal.

All of the sympathetic and parasympathetic responses we have been discussing are involuntary, or subconsciously controlled. In other words, you can't tell your digestive system to digest or not, nor can you tell your nerves how sensitive they should be. You can't put a finger on your pulse and through sheer willpower decide to change your heart rate from 72 beats per minute to 100.

But — and this is a big but — you can tell your respiratory system what to do.

You can, for instance, decide to change your respiratory rate from 20 breaths per minute to 10 breaths per minute. This is key to the human design because it gives us access to our autonomic nervous system. It gives us a key to the back door of how every other body system is regulated — and it is a skill that can be learned and mastered.

In Chapter 2, we will cover some of our favorite breathing and repositioning exercises.

CHAPTER 2: POSTURE

We The Asymmetrical

Are you symmetrical?

Take a peek in the mirror. If you have two arms and two legs, a nose in the middle, and ears on both side, you likely look symmetrical.

Consider Leonardo da Vinci's famed Vitruvian Man and you'll see what looks like a symmetrical human being.

But we are far from symmetrical.

Consider the liver. It's a large organ and it sits on the right side of our body. We have no liver on the left. The liver sits under the diaphragm and pushes it up, giving the right side leverage.

The heart sits towards the left side of our body, creating less room for the left diaphragm to move.

The diaphragm itself, the breathing muscle, is two to three times larger on the right side.[53]

Our left brain, which controls the right side of the body, is the analytical and more controlling side of the brain.[54]

The left side of the brain, which is more responsible for planning motion, controls the right side of the body. This creates an imbalance

---

[53] "Genetic specification of left–right asymmetry in the diaphragm muscles ...." 22 Jun. 2017, https://www.ncbi.nlm.nih.gov/pmc/articles/PMC5481184/. Accessed 21 Aug. 2018.

[54] "Left and Right Hemispheres - The Brain Made Simple." http://brainmadesimple.com/left-and-right-hemispheres.html. Accessed 27 Sep. 2018.

between right and left in terms of our proprioceptive awareness (where the body is in space) and our right-sided dominance.

We have three lobes of lung on the right and two on the left.

Although we look fairly symmetrical, there are numerous differences between the right and left side of our body.

We take 23,000 breaths per day. Every single time we breathe, because of the right-sided dominance of our diaphragm, there is a slight rightward pull of our spine and hips. We are constantly being pulled to the right all day long.

This biases us as humans towards the right side of our body. Because of this right-sided bias, we see a set of common muscle imbalances, positional issues, and patterns in the patients we treat.

These patterns are normal. Our body was designed with a larger diaphragm on the right and a tendency to pull rightward.

In a pre-Industrial Revolution world where we move often and with variety, these patterns are expressed in a healthy and normal manner.

But in our sedentary, little-moving society, these patterns become problematic. Like water running down a hill creates a larger groove over time, the patterns become more pronounced until we get to the point where tissues are being irritated by the way we are moving.

The Postural Restoration Institute,[55] or PRI, has done a great job of making sense of the common patterns we see in humans as a result of asymmetries. I'll lay them out below.

The Four Chains

The Brachial Chain (BC) influences movement of our neck, shoulder, and chest. It's comprised of muscles attached to the skull, scapula, and ribs. The brachial chain is opposed by the muscles in our back on the same side of the body.

The Anterior Interior Chain (AIC) influences our breathing, trunk rotation, and leg movements. This chain goes from the diaphragm all the way down to the knees.

The Posterior Exterior Chain (PEC) consists of the muscles on the back of our body from the top of the hips to the neck. These

---

[55] "PRI | Home." https://www.posturalrestoration.com/. Accessed 21 Aug. 2018.

chains of muscles act in opposition to the AIC and BC on the front of the body.

The Temporal-Mandibular-Cervical Chain (TMCC) is the muscles of the head and neck.

The Right Side Bias And Poor Breathing

As we mentioned earlier, we are set up to be drawn to the right side of our body. This, in combination with the stressful breathing we talked about in the last chapter, creates a common set of problems in most folks.

The rib cage in the front of the body is often flared up and in a poor position for breathing (usually more on the left)

The shoulder blades are in a poor position to provide stability and support for the arm (usually lower on the right).

The lower spine will rotate to the right with ease and the body will compensate by rotating back to the left.

There are numerous other compensations. What I want you to understand is not exactly how your body is in a poor position; rather, I want you to see the importance of position on creating the ability to move well.

Understand that shifting to the right side of our body was programed in us as a survival mechanism. It would have been important to not have to spend the milliseconds subconsciously thinking about which side of the body to use first thousands of years ago.

Shifting to the right side of our body is part of our sympathetic, stress-driven response. In our overly stressed society of today, this right-sided dominance has become more of a hindrance than a help.

Therefore, a common pattern of brain activity, breathing, and muscle activation is our body's way of promoting survival.

Why Does It Matter?

Let's discuss some of the practical ramifications of this right-side dominance when it's left unchecked.

Postures and movement patterns like the ones discussed above create asymmetries and sub-optimal movements in our joints, muscles, and connective tissues. Think of the person whose hip wears out at age 60 and they are told they have to get a hip replacement. Is this just bad luck or bad genes? No. It's probably due more to a poor and asymmetrical movement pattern.

If we can teach folks to change their movement patterns and to get to a state of neutrality, they will be much less likely to sustain wear and tear to their joints. No amount of painkillers or muscle relaxants can create neutrality.

With your body in a neutral or optimal position, you can safely know you're creating the "move well" communication you need in order to have long-lasting joints and a pain-free body.

From an athletic point of view, you'll never achieve your best performance if you are stuck in a sympathetic-driven, right-sided position. If your left rib cage is not in a position to take in air optimally, you won't be able to run or ride your bike for as far or as fast as possible. If you can't extend your left hip fully, you'll compensate by using less effective back extensors. This not only sets you up for injury but also makes you a less-than-optimal performer.

Exercises For Symmetry
See page 133 for Balloon Breathing and Wall Reach Exercise!

Why "Stand Up Straight" Is Bad Advice

We've worked with many who think that good posture means standing up very straight.

For most people, this means the flattened diaphragm, extended back, and hyperinflated chest associated with the fight-or-flight response.

Standing up straight makes good breathing impossible and does more harm than good.

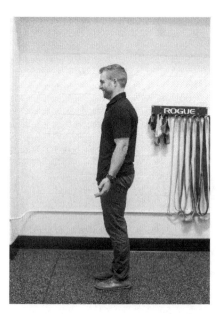

Here's a better way to stand. Stand up and do a full exhale. Pay attention to how your rib cage comes down. Then, try to hold your ribs in a slightly depressed position as you breathe. This will require you to activate your abs.

Your lower back should be relaxed.

Good posture should involve a slight rounding to our thoracic spine (upper back). This is counter to the current thinking in the health world today.

CHAPTER 3: UNDERSTAND PAIN

Pain As A Helper

Pain is meant to help us. Pain is meant to alert us to a potential threat. Pain is meant to move us towards action and change. Pain is normal.

Imagine walking across the living room and stepping on a tack. You'll quickly be alerted to the presence of the tack inside your toe by a jolt of pain. The pain prompts you to remove the tack from your toe and do important things like clean the wound. Without pain in this tack instance, you may not have noticed the tack. If left in your foot, the tack could do some serious tissue damage, cause infection, and potentially lead to the loss of the foot.

Pain Stories

Consider the paper cut. It's so small and the damage is so minimal, yet it hurts! Or how about those with phantom limb syndrome who have pain in their leg even though it has been amputated. On the other end of the spectrum, consider the person who has been wounded in combat, yet doesn't notice until after because they are so distracted with the battle at hand.

Take the story of a WWII vet who came in for a routine chest X-ray to find that he had a bullet lodged in his chest for the past 60 years and didn't even know it!

Pain Is Not Correlated With Tissue Damage

Many folks walk around with bulging discs, degenerative disc disease, and arthritis and feel no pain. Instead of making us fearful, this should give us hope.

Diagnoses like these are not a terminal sentence of pain and suffering for life.

The important thing to understand is that pain is labyrinthine and depends on many different factors. The brain determines whether or not we experience pain every single time.

Pain Depends On Context

If we think something will hurt, it's more likely to hurt. If we are shown a red light before a painful stimulus, more pain is likely to be experienced than if we see a blue light.[56]

I even noticed my son, Cooper, will look to me when he falls to see my reaction before he decides whether or not to cry.

The Alarm System

In PT school we read a book called *The Gift of Pain*. The book follows a medical doctor who worked with sufferers of leprosy overseas.[57]

People used to think that folks with leprosy lost limbs due to the disease itself. However, what we now know is that the disease causes destruction of the nerve endings responsible for sensation. This loss of sensation makes it difficult to detect sores on the feet, burns on the hands, and to ward off infections. The failure of the person with leprosy's alarm system is their demise.

We use memories, our eyes, our hearing, and our sense of smell to warn us of danger and protect us.

Imaging your body as a neighborhood. Each house is a small area of the body.

---

[56] "How the Color Red Influences Our Behavior - Scientific American." 1 Nov. 2014, https://www.scientificamerican.com/article/how-the-color-red-influences-our-behavior/. Accessed 27 Sep. 2018.
[57] "Gift of Pain, The: Paul Brand, Philip Yancey: 9780310221449: Amazon ...." https://www.amazon.com/Gift-Pain-Paul-Brand/dp/0310221447. Accessed 27 Sep. 2018.

Let's say the "knee house" is robbed. You tear your meniscus playing soccer and have a knee surgery. What would you do if your house was robbed? I bet you'd get some additional security systems, alert your neighbors, and be suspicious of anyone looking suspicious!

In the same way, your brain will go about protecting your knee. It will be more sensitive to pain from movements that did not used to be painful, and the areas around the knee may be painful.

Special Sensors

Inside our body, we don't have specialized sensors for pain. We have sensors for pressure, temperature, and even acid. What needs to happen for us to feel pain is for the brain to sense and perceive a threat.

Inside our brain a complex series of interactions takes place to determine if we will experience pain or not.

Hundreds of different parts of the brain are involved in the experience of pain.[58] There is not simply one area in the brain responsible for pain but rather a great, complex many working together.

The Brain's Orchestra

Imagine your brain as an orchestra. An orchestra can play an infinite number of different songs. Think of pain as one of those songs. When the pain tune is played over and over, it becomes difficult for the brain to play anything else.

The Communication Of Injury

When we are injured, we communicate with our body the need for repair. Thankfully, the human body is a really good healer. From bones to tendons to nerves, we can heal things. This is the time when inflammation is a good thing.

Pain is a normal part of this healing process and should decrease as tissues heal. Pain is there to protect us as we heal.

---

[58] "The Brain in Pain - NCBI - NIH."
https://www.ncbi.nlm.nih.gov/pmc/articles/PMC4405805/. Accessed 27 Sep. 2018.

Inflammation

Inflammation sensitizes our receptors in an area to increase perceptions of danger. When we eat a diet rich in sugar and vegetable oils and don't move often, this unchecked inflammation will increase our sensitivity to pain.

Understanding Is Empowering

Simply understanding pain can decrease the level of pain you feel.[59]

"Do you think the pain is in my head?" is a question I've often been asked by patients. Even though what they are really saying is "Do you think my pain is real?" I explain that all pain is processed and determined by our brains. But anyone who tells you your pain is not real is a quack!

Changes In The Alarm System

When we experience pain for long periods of time, the body and brain undergo adaptations.

Everything from our nerves, to our brain, and even our thoughts become more efficient at playing the pain tune.

Just like the orchestra that can only play the pain tune, your body get stuck. Strange things begin to happen. Some orchestra members may quit; others may tire of playing the same tune over and over again. The sound of the same song over and over again is not pleasant.

The increased alarm system on our recently robbed knee house is supposed to protect us from threats in the environment. But what if it was so sensitive that it went off every time a leaf blows by?

This is what happens when someone is in pain for a long time. When our brain becomes overly sensitive to stimuli even things normally not be painful like a touch on the skin, squatting, or running are perceived as threats. The alarm system is sounded and the pain tune continues to play.

---

[59] "Pain is Weird: A Volatile, Misleading Sensation - Pain Science." 26 Aug. 2018, https://www.painscience.com/articles/pain-is-weird.php. Accessed 27 Sep. 2018.

But There Is Hope

Thankfully, our nerves and brains have something called plasticity. This means they can change. Yes, it seems you can teach an old dog new tricks. At any age, given the right education and communication, you can signal your orchestra to begin to play a new tune (many new tunes!). You can turn down your alarm system and get back to doing the things you love.

1. First You Need Education And Understanding

Reread the section above. The book *Explain Pain* is an amazing resource as well.

Understand pain so it doesn't terrify you.

2. Pace Yourself

A few years ago, my wife was dealing with chronic knee pain every time she would ride her bike.

Each time we rode our bikes, she would start to get the pain at the 10-minute mark. Our rides were usually 50 minutes, so she would spend most of the ride in pain. This was feeding into the pain orchestra and allowing the tune to continue to play.

So I decided to encourage her to do something different. We went out for a five-minute bike ride. Yes, just five minutes. She didn't have any knee pain.

Later that week, it was eight minutes. And then 10. No pain. We were getting the orchestra to play a different tune. Slowly, minute by minute, we worked our way up to her riding for a full hour without knee pain. It was really cool!

Did we have some setbacks and flare-ups along the way? You bet! But it sure beat continuing to play the pain tune again and again.

3. Communicate Well With Your Body

Everything we've talked about leading up to this point in the book plays a role in your experience of pain. If you are always in an inflamed state, chronically stressed, and breathing poorly, you'll be more likely to have chronic pain.

Add to that the medications, surgeries, and current understanding of pain in our medical world, and it's a recipe for disaster.

Simply applying good nutritional and movement communication could be a major player in enabling you to live life pain-free.

4. See A Movement Specialist

There are many components of moving well that are far too nuanced to include in the pages of this book. I spent eight years getting educated to become a DPT and am constantly taking courses, reading, and learning.

Therefore, seeing someone in person is still the best way I can help them to move well.

If seeing us in our clinic at Village is not a possibility, find yourself a good physical therapist, chiropractor, or other movement specialist who will spend enough time with you to figure things out.

We spend an hour every session with our patients and even offer a free 30-minute consultation.

When I was working in the big healthcare system or insurance-based PT clinics, it was 15 to 25 minutes max. Everything about patients' care, from the appointment length to how often we could see a patient, was dictated by the insurance company.

Find someone who will work for you and not your insurance company.

CLOSING THOUGHTS

Investment

A few years ago, I purchased stock in the company Under Armour. They had just purchased My Fitness Pal, the calorie-tracking app I've recommended for the last six years, and they were on the rise.

As soon as I had invested in the stock, I started to notice and pay attention to all things Under Armour.

When someone would be wearing Under Armour clothes, I would stop and ask if they liked it. If I heard "Under Armour" in passing conversation, my ears perked up and I listened. When Under Armour was in the news, I paid attention. I even checked how the stock was doing about once a week.

I was invested in Under Armour.

Our bank accounts, credit card statements, or stock purchases show where our heart is.

The things we spend the most money on are the things we think about and care about most.

I didn't care about Under Armour's stock price (I didn't even know they were a publicly traded company) until the day I purchased the stock.

How we spend our hard-earned money is all about what we find value in.

If you value eating at nice restaurants and going on lavish vacations, you'll be willing to shell out cash for it.

If you value having a beautiful home, you'll spend on renovating the kitchen, making the backyard look nice, and nice decor. You can bet you'll spend a lot of time thinking about the home you've invested in.

If you value your health and being fit, you'll be more willing to spend money on gym memberships, healthy food, and personal training.

Invest more in the food you eat and your fitness coaching.

We live in a world where it's easy to grind away working up the corporate ladder. Before you realize it, you're in your 60s and retiring but riddled with chronic, preventable diseases, and every movement is painful.

But if folks invested in their health each and every month, it would occupy a larger area of brain space than it currently does in our culture.

Since I started doing all of the consulting with new clients at Village Fitness, I've encountered people who could not "afford" personal training because it was nearly as much as their car payment.

Sadly, these are folks who are generally in desperate need of personal training and nutrition coaching.

The big difference between a car and our body is that our body is guaranteed to last as long as we are alive. Your car is not.

Drive a car that you can pay cash for. Save your car payment for investing in your health. Here are some ideas.

It's important to put your money where you see value. If you pay for a healthy meal delivery service or personal training sessions, you're going to show up. The results you seek will take care of themselves.

If you let culture dictate how you spend your money, you'll end up taking nice vacations and driving a sweet car, but you'll likely be overweight, unhealthy, and not able to do the things you want to do long-term.

When you invest your money into something you believe in, you're more likely to make it a reality.

Be Curious
"The world is full of magical things patiently waiting for our senses to sharpen." - Not-Sure-Who

Cooper, my son, has recently discovered the letter E. Although he has about a 75% success rate at finding it, when he does, he gets excited and proclaims "EEEE!"

His eyes light up, get wide, and his face brightens as he is learning and forming the connections between letters and the world. It's pretty cool.

It makes me appreciate the little things and makes me want to get clients excited about the food they eat and the movement they do.

If our only motive for exercise is to lose weight, it makes the process of losing weight a chore. If we are constantly restricting the food we eat in an effort to look a little better or have less body fat, it creates guilt around our eating experience.

Instead, recognize that everything you need to live a healthy, lean, pain-free life is already programmed into your DNA. How amazing is that?

Be curious. Be a lifelong learner. Devour the lessons we put out, ask good questions on our coaching calls, and be an active participant in the vibrant community of Village.

Focus on the process, and the results will take care of themselves.

There is much joy to be had in the process of discovering and learning to appreciate the little things in our food and movement.

The food we eat and the movement we do are like a language that communicates with our DNA.

ABOUT THE AUTHORS

Dr. Matt Klingler is a physical therapist and the owner of Village. He has a vision for Village to become a comprehensive solution for helping people optimize their health and live pain-free, vibrant lives. He and his wife, Nicole, have two amazing kids, Cooper and Chloe.

Dr. Erik Gullen is a creative genius. He does amazing things with his manual therapy skills, knowledge of the human body, and love for people. He is a doctor of physical therapy. He and his wife, Krissy, live in Glendora.

Made in the USA
Columbia, SC
19 August 2024

40254879R00105